THE RUNNING JOURNEY

ALI MAZHIN

PAGE PUBLISHING
Conneaut Lake, PA

First originally published by Page Publishing 2022

ISBN 978-1-6624-8656-2 (pbk)
ISBN 978-1-6624-8657-9 (digital)

Printed in the United States of America

The story that I'm writing is about my running journey that started at a young age and continues onto today. Running is a process of terrestrial locomotion letting humans and other animals to move rapidly on foot.

I remember as an infant in Iran in 1979 that there were various people around me as my mom held me while I listened and saw my surroundings. My relatives were living at different nearby houses while they helped one another finish their work. The sounds of the neighborhood and sight of windows at the housing complexes were vivid and broadcasted a series of light sounds as I envisioned life being very unique.

I had the cognitive ability to contemplate as a young baby. Today, many adults live their lives in competition as they race toward an imperfect goal often forgetting how they felt in preschool. The activity of running lets me envision success in many areas to find myself reach higher goals and feel happier with existence.

The memory of my surroundings was distinctive because the technological culture of Iran differs from America. My family communicated at an intelligent level because their culture was strong and affectionate. I enjoyed hugging and playing and doing normal activities similar to most people, and success seemed to be in reach because I wanted to be happy. My senses felt a wave of pressure that often make people smile or frown, similar to waves of plasma or lava that move in the outside world.

The wave of thinking made me realize how I view other people as well-thought-of individuals. When I go running, the feelings become a natural sense of enjoyment because my mind is active while

I realize others on my route. My mental effort and vision let me communicate to other people that smile and live a normal lifestyle.

The illustrations of growing up as a kid to an adult show me that in a race, you don't need to worry about faster runners ahead of you, but instead focus on quickness for each mile, one at a time without burning out. At the starting line of a race, line up at the right spot, and the faster runners are at the front, and the slower runners are in the back. Oftentimes, you're standing at the start, which shows you're ready to run and use your body, energy, and muscle movement to move in stride safely. Once you pass someone, you can have an instant glory and remember back your favorite childhood spot.

In Iran, my late grandmother and other relatives always held me to let me see how I'd smile, and the culture in Iran was changing rapidly with the Revolution. My relatives were happy in Iran, but my parents decided to leave after the Revolution in 1979 to have better lives in America. My father got accepted to study for a PhD program in accounting at Indiana University Bloomington, and I have memories of walking with my father on campus and in the halls as he made time for me to talk with his colleagues and faculty and let me feel assured.

Most people are not sharp enough to view or taste success early in life and actually live it later, but you can make your journey work by using your available resources.

My journey started when I was young with many kids my age and professional teachers let us ride tricycles, rest together, and play, which made me enjoy the outdoors. I rode my bike in preschool and remembered seeing my father come to pick me up with a smile because I made efforts to be energetic.

The state of Indiana left me to envision as a child how to stand on my feet when others were around. Crawling as a baby was a way to hold my head upright and look at how my family lived in their generation with many friends and a cat. They lived lives that stood apart from others because they were happy and successful. My father took my family and me for car rides, and he used to often smoke cigarettes through the many turns around mountains in his BMW.

Through communication, I learned independence, to feel I was capable of trying new things and to set attainable goals

My father was realistic in how to raise a family for me to have my own perceptive, qualities, and characteristics that made me stand out from others. I wouldn't get taken advantage of, and I would learn to grow and make sense of my own characteristics. Today, I carried my love into participating in running events to feel a sense of purpose and trust my decisions are made with good judgment. In today's world, you must focus on the present and be aware and mindful of what's going on at this moment instead of being distracted to keep your attention on your interests.

Upon moving to California from Indiana in 1982, after my sister was born, my experiences with sports and entertainment grew. The Olympics had many running events and athletes in other events that were fascinating to view and follow. My elementary school was called Silver Spur, and I ran near the red-and-white school poles with others between classes. I often hung out by myself near the roof of the school, and my mind became stronger and pushed me to grasp the idea that isolation did not feel normal.

The physical activity of dodgeball and handball were normal, and I kept up with most kids. There were also book sales and ice cream socials, and I was able to talk with family and friends about my progress as a kid and the sports I loved. The car rides I had early in life brought me to stand more on the ground today.

The start of intermediate school was at Malaga Cove and later at Palos Verdes Intermediate, and my picture came in the class yearbook and read "Crazy legs." I was always active and my legs went places, and some unhealthy choices happened after that time.

The only sport that I tried out for was my high school basketball team at Palos Verdes Peninsula High School, but I did not make the team, and I saw the intensity of other athletes. In physical education or PE, there was a running event where I enjoyed passing the baton to the other runners around the high school track. Other sports such as roller-skating, skateboarding, hockey games, paintball games, golf, swimming, badminton, tennis, softball, baseball, ice-skating, ice hockey, weight lifting, and lacrosse kept me absorbed in sports.

Today, cycling has profound effects on many people's lives to stay active. The 24 Hour Fitness gym, which is a privately owned fitness center chain with headquarters in Carlsbad, California, is where I often cycled in classes, and I gained flexibility, and I used it for running. Running is an efficient form of exercise for burning calories, and it burns more calories than cycling, and your body uses more muscles. Running requires less equipment than other sports and brings out deeper emotions to perform your best. The sport of indoor cycling needs the athlete to focus on seeing the classroom, listening to the instructor, and staying levelheaded.

The news, media, and television discuss how the world changes because of the COVID-19 pandemic and how it affects people in different ways, including symptoms, precautions, or ways to avoid getting sick. The COVID-19 pandemic stopped indoor cycling momentarily at my local gym in Torrance, but as a runner, I found a way to get out on a marathon course or a virtual course that led me to increase running. By participating in various running series and events such as Series Runner that moves runners in the right direction, I found that it keeps me just as busy as my primary physician, and I focus on enjoying life more with activities that make various challenges worthwhile.

The body naturally repairs and restores tissue damaged from your workout and releases human growth hormone (HGH) with more sleep. My body was exercising more than sleeping for a bit of time, and I've found tremendous progress toward better sleep.

I handed the COVID-19 pandemic well because when businesses and my local gym closed, I reframed to create new goals in running. Before the pandemic, I would spend about two to five hours exercising in the gym on a Sunday morning, starting with a cycle or spin class; a BODYPUMP class, which is a barbell class; a BODYCOMBAT class, which is a mixed martial art workout; and a yoga class for relaxation after. I would visit the gym at least twice on a Sunday and go to a yoga class in the evening and then run on the treadmill for almost four hours for endurance for my races.

In the gym, there are different settings to choose on a treadmill that help to be more running minded. Once people exercise together, there is a wind that blows that felt similar to how your perception of your life is seen from within. Similar to when someone is in high school or another school, the student tries to feel accepted within groups of people while time is on their side. When a person leaves this setting or graduates, they are put in a special group, or they can be classified as graduates.

The local 24 Hour Fitness gym had the fastest runners watching television side by side on the treadmill who were said to have completed the Boston Marathon. I first trained on the treadmill with a similar passion and at a level that was faster than most.

My running and productivity improved during the time the COVID-19 pandemic shut down the government in March 2020, as the pandemic lessened more places opening for business. I was naturalized and became a US citizen in my teens, but in Iran, my birth records were misplaced because of the Iranian Revolution. My parents tried to get my date of birth record straight, but my birthday today in America is right and differs from my Iranian calendar birth date. The United States is the land of opportunity because a large amount of people left their homes to come full circle or for an opportunity to succeed. I can view the full circle of success that running has given me, and I live with many cultures of people in the United States.

The ultimate goal when training for a marathon is to run at a faster pace and advance your finish time to qualify for a different race. The Boston Marathon or Western States are races that are more difficult to qualify for, but by focusing on a goal of having enjoyable runs and a stronger body, it's worthwhile. Completing various challenges provided by a marathon can be exciting once you get more medals. I was living my life to be unique, and it set myself apart from others to get ahead or to feel distinctive as a whole.

With more training, the body can be move well and experience the positive effects of the exercise such as losing weight or lowering your risk of heart disease. The mind-body connection can work to your advantage and allow you to run fast, save energy, and be flexible by utilizing areas of your body that haven't been used before. Being ready to run can give the sense of happiness, and if you start at a slow pace, you can pick it up later, but if you run throughout the whole race, you build confidence with your mood.

Many people who dream in life have so-called nightmares because they set their expectations too high. A goal of many runners is to feel comfortable in their daily lives outside of their runs. I'm able to reach further for a goal of an adequate pace because I'm flexible to let my body recover. There are many people in life that try to work hard and have the mindset to be healthier, but with running, they can reach their goals and find a balance that makes them happy. The healthier person has an advantage while running because they are more content with themselves and fit. By learning more about running, I've been able to view race websites and learn more about challenges and appreciate the simplicity of training and take the steps needed to run healthier.

Runners that train and participate in events together can set attainable goals, and you can vision yourself running faster and living life stronger. Runners improve their pace during runs by believing in themselves and finding ways to keep a constant pace throughout the race. Runners I meet at races who run with a faster pace than me can feel as though I outperformed them when we talk at the finish line because of the number of marathons I've run.

Runners improve their pace due to many factors such as eating healthy, exercising, having family well-being, or having better mental health. One way running motivates me is to run within the rules of various challenges because I know I'm part of something greater than the race. Since I'm grateful for my health, I experience joy when running, and I give myself credit for it. Running also has social media websites to follow and use such as Twitter, Facebook, and Instagram, and there are options that let you post your time and selfie picture online for others to see.

My first marathon was the San Francisco Marathon in 2008, and my training program was with the National AIDS Marathon training program in Los Angeles. An old friend of mine talked to me into signing up for the program through a flyer at a local donut shop. I started to fundraise toward the minimum goal, and I trained with a group of runners for about six months in Griffith Park, and it was amazing because I grew into a successful runner. The AIDS Marathon training program is now closed, but they helped me to push myself to a higher stage in running, and I met many people.

My weight was about 270 pounds before starting the training program, and today my weight is consistent at about 163. The proper way to make a life change is to focus on the whole picture and feel proud of your accomplishments. Set goals that are realistic, and look back and feel after you achieve the goal that the change is permanent and a part of you. Running can make a person stronger by going back to the basics to see what your lifestyle was missing. I always enjoy my birthday parties because I can eat cake, get presents, talk with friends, be with family, and it's only one day a year, and I've often passed on cake because it can make me feel guilty later.

A running partner can help you achieve your goals faster. The 2007 San Francisco Aids Marathon training program helped me find a consistent schedule to train with groups of people. I listened my running buddies I met during the training program who pushed, encouraged, and supported me from the first day of training until to the end of the race. In Griffith Park, the two coaches, Tim and Dave, often used a microphone in the morning to motivate the runners into assigned groups for two- to nine-mile weekly runs. They underlined, "It's a feeling that lasts a lifetime" or how good you'll feel after completing the marathon.

There were goodies such as pretzels, water, juice, and sweets to eat after each run on a bench and table provided by the runners and coaches, which was satisfying. In an actual marathon, the treats on the course are often water, drinks with electrolytes such as Gatorade, protein bars, cookies, Cheez-Its, fruit, energy shots, and even beer. In my situation, after learning the basics of running, I slowly began to race and register for races on my own, which made me feel professional.

I flew to San Francisco with my dad in 2007, and I was influenced to run by people I remembered who were ice-skaters or ice hockey players. By routing my motivation to running, which was simpler and easier to learn than most sports, I had the opportunity to compete with others in a friendly manner.

In the 2007 San Francisco Marathon, I sent my former employer, owner of the Redbrick Pizza, a text message, saying, "I'm on the Golden Gate Bridge running a marathon." This message isn't something I'd write today, but it did come to me at a time when I was traveling to the Golden Gate Bridge and seeing the roads blocked off in a way that I felt an urge to share my joy with someone that I knew.

Although I got no response, since I was running a marathon, I had a sense of comfort knowing that event staff and volunteer people of the race would not take my messaging the wrong way because of the excitement I was feeling at that time. I found my discipline to be there for me to succeed and finish my first marathon.

The structure of graduate school eight years later was the breaking point in my running because I was surrounded by gifted students in my business classes that made some of my classes dream classes.

I don't drink alcohol anymore because I'm past my party days, which provided little satisfaction and social acceptance. I decided to temporarily bring my own protein bars during races, which helped me to be less hungry.

The 2017 Los Angeles Marathon offered complimentary Clif shots before the race, and I had too many, which put me in the hospital at night with dehydration, gastritis, colitis, rhabdomyolysis, ileus, abdominal pain, and gastroenteritis. When your muscles cramp and start to feel fatigued, you have the options of either giving your full energy level, not giving up, acknowledging you have the pain but run through it, or you can quit the race.

I had a choice to stop and give up during my 2017 Los Angeles Marathon, but I choose not to give up and finish the race. After the eighth or ninth mile, I began to vomit because my stomach could not handle the blocks. While my muscles felt cramped and fatigued, it became harder for me to finish the race, and it took me almost ten hours to finish. My body knew its limits, but I kept going. I learned not to eat too many caffeine energy blocks and to stay hydrated. I actually had about ten packages of Clif caffeine energy blocks before the race, and my body did not want to take it.

After the race, when getting to my bed, my stomach had an empty feeling and I needed to vomit more. I got dehydrated, and one of my kidneys nearly failed, so I went to the emergency room at the local hospital and stayed as an inpatient for seven days. There were many tests given to me to discover the reason for my abdominal pain, and it seemed to be from the running and the way my body had cramps from the food I ate. The journey of being able to build my health for the better has been ongoing, and it is helping me today to deal with the stresses of everyday life, such as when people tell me that I lost a lot of weight or of how to feel better from misunderstanding people's comments.

With the support of my parents, relatives, and classmates, I was able to make it out on time for my group presentation in my finance class at California State University Dominguez Hills (CSUDH). I spent my time wisely in the hospital studying my finance book and studying and writing papers for my other course in Strategic Management. I remember the days I was absent from my class, and it was interesting because after perfect attendance for nearly one year and half, I missed two classes. I also had a nurse write me two notes to send to my professors so they would understand that I was out of class for a medical reason in my masters of business administration (MBA) program. I was able to recover from rhabdomyolysis, ileus, abdominal pain, acute kidney injury, gastroenteritis, and dehydration.

Now that I look at how many of my classmates and I are still friends, I can see the reality of how important it is to attend your classes when you can. Many classmates were also absent from classes when they didn't feel well, so I understood myself.

In today's work setting and working world at my job at Ralphs, I can see that many people have different perceptions as to how management is run. For example, the management at Ralphs is managing me to do work that is needed and to get people to fill in their shifts when it is needed.

A healthy diet and continuous exercise schedule keep me fit during all times. The biggest obstacle that I overcame was getting dehydrated during the 2017 LA Marathon, but it was overcome by changing my diet and exercise, and the most rewarding part of my training is being able to take rests. Medals given after races and making it home safe is rewarding. Keep as close to running your assigned miles per week with your training schedule as possible either online or with a trainer. A healthy diet and exercise routine can improve your chances of performing sound in a marathon. The opportunity to participate in various online training programs helped me to build my running skills immensely because it gave me a clear path about a number of miles each week, either at the gym or in the neighborhood.

Most marathons runners have a common goal to run the race in a certain time limit, improve health, or to qualify for the Boston Marathon. To qualify for the Boston Marathon, a runner needs to be at least eighteen years of age and need to race in a certified full-length marathon taking place within a year of the Boston Marathon and then report your qualifying race and time. For me to qualify for my age group of forty to forty-four, my qualifying standard time is three hours, ten minutes, and zero second; and my qualification time accepted is three hours, eight minutes, and twenty-one seconds.

Runners gain a perspective on how to train for a marathon with their thoughts. The varying lifestyles of runners also plays a part on how they adapt to the challenges and pleasures they see on the course. Increasing pace near the end of the race has helped me to perform well, and it can be done with confidence, control, and collection to prevent yourself from collapsing or feeling pain.

My experience of running several races shows me that even though I haven't qualified to run the Boston Marathon, I can piece together certain moments in races that I've performed well in and see how and where I can improve. Also, in 2020, and in 2021 there was a Virtual option for the Boston Marathon that makes it a more attainable goal. Virtual runs let you learn more about running and racing in person to finish. I trained at the gym with an old friend that inspired me to see what it takes to run the Boston Marathon because he knew how to train effectively, but safety was the key. A way to make this work is to envision yourself while you are running at the gym as if you were outside running in a race, mile after mile.

Oftentimes, qualifying for the Boston Marathon can be similar to making it in the big leagues of baseball. A person can try so hard for the goal, but the chances of actually achieving can be slim. To actually push your body to the standards of the top athletes, there are some lifestyle changes that must be made. For me, in March of 2017, I started to follow a diet with less processed meats and an exercise routine that matched my goals, and I lost about sixty-five pounds.

Even though you are not physically at a race, your mental energy can be similar to what it's like in a race. With an idea of how to keep pace during a run, you will see reactions in others because you're more comfortable in your running. It can be thrilling to set a new goal such as qualifying for the Boston Marathon because of the course reputation. Since I want to run the Boston Marathon, I feel that the virtual marathon would be an entertaining experience because people who run the marathon need to train year-round to be healthy enough to finish. Recovering mentally and physically after a marathon doesn't have to feel like work, and you can regain energy later and make healthier choices.

Exercise can help you lessen fatigue, lower stress, and lessen work absences and make time in your day to run. The vigor that running brings you on a course have a different feeling when exercising because it can be a challenge if your body aches up. The help from others besides you can motivate you last throughout the race. In a public place such as the gym, there are many people exercising in a facility, and that is where I have spent large amounts of time trying to train better for runs when today I can see that I was often overtraining.

Running can be a channel to grow through keeping a mindset of more physical activity for the prize after the next race. The journey of living happily and rest are experienced by many. For example, people who work at a gym wear name tag or a bagger at a grocery store shows his name and what he loves, and you can feel you are in the right place, greeted by a service representative. This feeling of peacefulness comes in my communication at the gym or a grocery store with many types of cardiovascular equipment to see and ideas to eat a balanced diet. Many people lift weights and attend classes and let people guide them, similar to going through a grocery store and walking through the aisles with making better choices in diet. Before a marathon, you have been given feedback by many people at the gym, work, and other places where people greet you and talk to you. Once you start your course, you try to run a fast pace to the finish line.

The time spent in a gym can be exhausting on the mind and body even before you get to the gym, and if you have fatigues, your muscles tire quickly, which means you need to get rest to see the benefits gradually on your body.

The gym has a front desk that makes you feel welcome, where they answer phones, questions, help with preparing classes, and keep the area clean. I found the time to work, earn money, and I let my body decide whether it's better to run or participate in a facility, and I chose to run more.

Oftentimes at my local club, I felt that I was the only one that had a strong vision of work, ethic, and goals, but many others have them too. By seeing a few people at my job at Ralphs, which is an American supermarket chain in Southern California and largest subsidiary of Kroger, and later working as a delivery driver with Postmates before it was bought by Uber Eats, I make smarter purchases. Uber Eats is an online food ordering and delivery platform made in 2014 by Uber, where customers read menus and reviews, order, and pay for food from restaurants using their phone app, and they often tip for delivery.

The gym had an environment unlike any other place that made me enjoy being a member. Once I canceled my membership, I found an app called Future that worked with 24 Hour Fitness that has just as many benefits as the gym without having to go there. The monthly dues of the gym in Torrance had a number of amenities such as personal training, the store, and some classes, which could be expensive, and I became comfortable with my achievements outside of the gym and made a plan to get good workouts and run without going to the gym.

Running stories can be told in many ways, and my story of running starts with how I learned from my mistakes as I grew, I created goals, and later trended toward a journey of success through running various races. I learned what my body needed to stay healthy to complete 295 races to date, 82 of which were marathons. Consistency in training, a healthy diet, enough rest, and access to experienced coaches with online training who can continue to guide me along the way have helped me to win. My secret to success is to, at some time in your life, get as much training as possible for every marathon and train whenever and however you can or want.

I saw the world as whole, a series of choices and events where I had individuality and manners to make ends meet. As an athlete, it can be a learning experience to go through the sequence of events that lead to me to run a marathon such as to find a race, register, go to the expo, run, and recover. For example, I had a job at Elite Development Enterprises, and my work was as an account manager and assurance wireless representative. The company had an eight- to twelve-month management training program. It could seem to be the same amount of physical work as the life of the busiest athlete in the world because of working on improving to sell the company's product and produce more.

In running events, you can learn more about yourself, be flexible, and where you are in life and how to get the next level. When the idea of running comes to mind, my first thought is physical exertion because I'm using my body's energy to run at a pace to get to a new point.

I learned in my last three months working as an account manager at Elite Development Enterprises that I can still train my body for a marathon without the countless hours that I used to spend at the gym. GX classes, running on the treadmill, weight lifting, swimming, and cardiovascular exercises kept me in shape today. With the opportunity to recently still visit the gym four to six times a day or night and adapting to the notion, it made me figure out a new way to train my body for running and to set myself up for future success. The gym experience varies from actual marathon running because at the race you're is in a different environment, and you need to be smarter about using the porta potties. You don't want to pee on yourself. Volunteers try to give praise and encouragement to help you make changes toward a faster marathon and a better style.

The difference in seeing your finish time and seeing someone else's time in a marathon can keep you motivated. When a runner reads about the runner who placed first in a marathon, they are able to sense that possibility of improving their time or win an award in their age division. It could seem far-fetched to earn first place, but if you know that someone placed well in their race then you can try just as hard to find a way to win. The successful figures in the business world often build a fortune on their own and leave you to make that similar attempt to succeed.

During my 2018 San Francisco Marathon, I had an unusual experience after the twentieth mile where I was led to believe I was winning the race. I was running the race on pace and felt that I was doing well as the volunteer told me that I was winning the race and pointed where I should run. I listened and acknowledged the volunteers and kept my pace to finish strong. There were some people running alongside me, but by the time I crossed the finish line, I asked the volunteers about a special award for winning the race because the volunteer told me I was winning.

The volunteers at the finish line tent agreed with me and told me to send an email to the San Francisco Marathon staff and tell them what the volunteers said in regard to me winning the race. The San Francisco Marathon staff got back to me and told me that what the volunteers said was not true. They triple-checked the results and did not decide to mail me an Age Division Award, but they did mail me another 40 for 40 Challenge medal.

My ambitions to improve my repertoire grew as I became more confident in researching various marathon topics and how to run better. I decided to sign up for the 2019 San Francisco Ultramarathon, and by training at the gym for seven to eight hours a day, I became ready to run and finish the race with a fast time.

In running longer distances such as ultramarathon, the runner usually competes with runners from across the United States in ultrarunning or ultradistance. When signing up for these races longer than marathons with mileage from above 26.2 to 200 miles, the runner registers by inputting their information such as their name, distance, and the city they live in for the race roster to be complete.

The most common ultramarathons are 50K, 50 miles, 100K, and 100 miles. When I register on UltraSignup, I enter my city as

Rancho Palos Verdes and later see the list of runners from all different areas. I know there's a world of runners to meet that come from many nations. The feeling of being well prepared and healthy lets me choose carefully to find well-organized races that are worthwhile.

The San Francisco Ultramarathon itself was a little bit challenging because I was not used to some of the operating guidelines. There was a speech by the race director Michael Li in the Hyatt before the race where he said how to use the restrooms during the first marathon, lap, or loop.

I used the emergency contacts on my cell phone and kept pushing throughout the race to help me finish the first marathon with a satisfactory time. It became easy to get lost and veer off the course because it seemed as though I was on my own, with the limited number of sixty-eight runners, we tried to stay in packs and run throughout the race. There was an app called RunGo that the staff let the runners know to download that showed which way to go during the course. It helped me finish.

The finish line in a double marathon or ultramarathon can seem different for a runner, but in San Francisco, you are actually finishing the race with the runners who signed up for the 26.2-mile marathon, where some completed a marathon and others completed two. In the finish line for the San Francisco Ultramarathon, I felt positive as the runners and I walked together to the appropriate tent and area to get our double marathon medals.

In finishing the ultramarathon, I spoke to various runners about how much training and effort I put into the race, which made me feel as if I was in my own state of mind after exercising in various classes at the gym, when I'm far away from my home to the gym. Some classes at the gym had members that started at different times than the class started and the level of intensity changed to feel unclear, but my viewpoint was to make myself feel justified for being able to keep myself healthy and experience life.

At home, often after long hours of work, there are time that my body gets so tired in front of my computer that I need to sleep. I can feel the help that some of the effects exercises and my running had given me. The concept of time being relative to everyone as people work and feel life as genuine humans is similar to a stranger in a strange land needing to adapt to the civilization.

Upon finishing my ultramarathon, my barriers of communication broke as I met others who traveled from other countries to enjoy a meal. Family life at home and social life at the gym brought me to where I was. After the ultramarathon, the word *Embarcadero* was seen again, and it showed the scenery changes for a clear view ocean with sunshine with the street in a brighter light. In a beautiful place such as the Embarcadero, which is where the race started, had many runners together with volunteers at 5:30 a.m., preparing for the start waves of the runners. With seeing so many runners and people getting ready for the race and the feedback the volunteers gave me, there's a sense of readiness to have a great run and to feel the energy of the marathon staff.

After running the race in two laps, with the first lap being run in reverse, a runner can now see how the trees, ocean, and city has made that area a famous place with it being one of the most beautiful marathons next to Boston. A person can now feel appreciation for the people that they see on a regular basis such as a gas station attendant, a grocery clerk, a cashier, a gardener, a school teacher, a parent, or a loved one.

Los Angeles International Airport is the main international airport serving Los Angeles and its surrounding metropolitan areas as many tourists come and go from different countries that can give me a social image of how runners throughout the world travel. When a person goes to LAX, you must use your time to socialize to understood where to go and use the television with terminals as a guide. When my return from San Francisco came after the ultramarathon in 2019, I felt an instant boost of confidence with my mom as she picked me up from the airport and drove me home because I was relaxed and saw the world in a better perspective. By remembering family that supports before and after the run, there are more pluses that you'll remember in your marathon.

In perspective, oftentimes, it is said that a business student is a person that can get the ground running at some point in their lives by taking proper study tools to pass the GMAT exam. A student who studies for the GMAT exam can, for example, be prepared to score higher if they purchase certain study material by GMAC to get a higher score on their exam.

It can also be said that some astronauts will today escape COVID-19 by traveling outside the earth. In an article written by Series Runner about me in 2020, the headline read, "Runner escapes COVID-19," meaning that with all of my twenty races toward the series, it enabled me to bypass the stigma and illness of COVID-19. With these examples of how special people can achieve extraordinary feats and later make the world a better place for themselves and others, it can be said that runners can, at some time, join an area of people in society that distinguishes them from others.

In my experience I have also taken the GMAT exam myself and performed well, enough to make it into a business school at California State University Dominguez Hills and also graduate at the top of my class with a master in business administration with the only campus major general business.

When I graduated from CSUDH, I went to my sister's old house and felt a feeling of accomplishment, which was a moment that was enjoyed with family. When a lifetime of energy has been put into graduation from graduate school, a family member was there to reflect and let me remember the experience. Similar to running and after completing a marathon, there is a time to enjoy with family afterward.

After graduating high school, I enrolled in El Camino Community College, and I adapted to many changes in my schedule. I drove to class at the junior college to get there by 8:00 a.m. and noticed it was easy to get sidetracked in my car ride as friends telling me stories on the telephone at home about El Camino. It prepared me to learn how to think differently and to feel in place. A characteristic that made me feel successful was that I can go to school with a calm attitude. I tried not to question the paths that many others have taken or not to compare myself and set a clear path in school to help me to stay physically and mentally healthy. Similarly, when running a marathon there is a lot of information given to you such as the starting point, an announcer that discusses the weather, prizes, the course, the race itself, and the finish line party, which can give you enough incentive to want to perform well in your run.

In actual marathons, the finish line party is a place where you can feel accomplished and enjoy the time. The finish line party at some marathons costs money to join, but the majority of them are free with the race. There are special massages you can get, special types of food to help you recover better, and special items given to you from the race at the party. Oftentimes in VIP areas, there are places where you can eat healthy food. The finish line party of events can be looked at as a positive experience to celebrate your achievement.

One thing that can help you in your journey is making a vision for yourself that there is a clear-cut path to the finish line or a clear set of characteristics that help most runners follow and finish. The more you put into your runs with proper training, communication, feedback, and discipline, the faster and smarter you can run. My path includes many hours of training, social interaction, and work to improve myself as a person too. I started going to California State University Dominguez Hills as an undergraduate with a major in business administration with an emphasis in finance, and I knew the social impact and time exercise has on others and what it brought to the classes I attended. A good value is that whatever time you put into running or any other form of exercise, it usually pays off in one way or another, especially if you have a proper diet and exercise regimen to follow. Communication throughout your run to properly pass others is similar to working harder to make pain-free and smarter decisions.

The first time I started to body build by lifting weights was at the age of seventeen where I counted the calories I ate and included protein shakes and meal replacement bars in my diet. In addition, I ate at El Pollo Loco for some meals. Educational goals also let me ponder health goals such as improving my muscle size, and I was on a path to victory.

Often, wanting to accomplish more and more is common, and while a marathon runner actually runs his or her mindset, it's usually set on maintaining a comfortable pace mile after mile. The fastest and best runners train with 70–180 miles of running per week nearby their homes. My average week running has had me run about 80 miles or sometimes closer to 30 if it becomes more of a work week.

The next phase of my life after graduating with my undergraduate degree in finance from California State University Dominguez Hills was being able to find some work that gave me experience in the business field to manage my money better. My dad had a CPA firm called Tax Advice Inc. that helped me gain experience by working with an accounts payable secretary. I met various clients of my dad on a daily basis and accomplished many accounting and finance tasks for his firm through Microsoft Excel.

If you are in an office all day long, it could seem as though you are not moving enough, but with proper stretching and walking and financing your money well, you can move as much as your body wants to go. My ability to register for various marathons at work was a way for me to actually see how a lot of businesses are run because many marathons have sponsorships with other businesses. Along with the registration fees for a race, I learned that with race registration protection, you can protect your registration fee in case there's an illness or injury and you are not able to run on race on the day.

A choice to continue running marathons was made after my first marathon in San Francisco. The various marathons that I choose to run were on Long Beach, Surf City, Orange County, Palos Verdes, Ventura, and Los Angeles, all of which were located in California and were well-liked races.

The Long Beach Marathon was the closet race to me, and it combines remarkable oceanfront views, attractive seaside communities, and an urban feel at the start and finish line. The experience of running through the California State University Long Beach (CSULB) campus was electrifying because by having a road map of how marathons were structured, I enjoyed running through a school and studying the architecture.

The courses of each marathon differ while some are more difficult than others because of hills, and others have more scenery, making them enjoyable. If you love sport stars or academics, try to keep and think of them as your heroes while running, and it can be pleasurable and motivating throughout the race and later in your daily life. I like various trees, scenery, the ocean, academics, work, sport stars, and the architecture of various houses. While running a race, there are many forms of nature to see, and the environment along the course can make you appreciate everything yourself to have gratitude.

The Long Beach Marathon is one of the marathons that I have the longest streak for. I've run it every year since 2009, and in 2019, I was recognized by the marathon staff for running ten years in a row. I was given a special medal commemorating ten years as a Beach Bum. It might sound a little odd to be labeled a Beach Bum after continuously running a 26.2-mile race, but to get the recognition, you should be in the Beach Bum club, which is a legacy club. The Long Beach Marathon volunteers often give me feedback along the course, and when I am getting close to the finish line, I feel excited to finish with a smile. Once I'm running past miles twenty-two and twenty-four, I usually can find ways to finish stronger because I see my purpose in running the race even though I might be exhausted.

Some running professional are sponsored and place in the top three of their events, as they enjoy the sport without getting carried away. Oftentimes, the biggest races give me the appreciation being with professional runners, and after the event, I hang my medals in my room, advance in the various challenges, and collect shirts or other items that show my accomplishment.

A balance of feeling good with your family, hobbies, and meeting people when you run and a comfortable living with work can make you happy instead of focusing on goals that are not attainable. The legacy clubs in various marathons can make you feel just as comfortable as some of the most successful people because you have time to enjoy being with an exclusive set of runners. The journey of feeling good can start with your decision listening to perspectives of others after your race and retaining pleasant memories to run or exercise to.

Many times, there is daylight savings changes before you've had your run, and you adjust your time with confidence; and after your run, you go back to normal life or work routine and see the harder part is over and you've grown to feel mentally and physically stronger.

By being in various legacy clubs such as the Surf City Marathon Long Board Legacy Club, you are being recognized by the race that you have participated in for three years. By adding things in your life such as work goals, improving yourself physically, you can feel balanced and well. Running can be something in your life that helps you meet goals if you plan carefully without over exhaustion or overtraining yourself. The feeling I had oftentimes with too much exercise to train for races was that I wanted to get more sleep, and it was not easy to do, but I made it work by changing my routines. In today's times, with challenges of various diseases, people know to be careful to live a long and healthy life.

The Surf City Marathon is one of the best courses in the country and is mostly flat, and many people are in running clubs and loyalty programs. The Long Board Legacy Club is a special club that lets its members enjoy the benefits after three years of running either full or half marathons. The prize is usually a T-shirt that can be given before the race, and after the race, you are granted access to the beer garden, but since I do not drink alcohol, it is seldom attended. There used to be an emblem that you can put on your medal, which shows your status in the club.

After a race is over, there are often many runners that stay connected through online training, social media, or even legacy clubs. This type of friendship can let a person reap the benefits of their run and often be congratulated. The discussions of the various key points of the race with others can make the finish line experience better improved. I usually ask runners how their time and experience was in their run. I almost always get a positive response from the runners because they congratulate me on my run and tell me it's nice to meet them.

The Surf City Marathon has a Kona Brewing Longboard legacy club where the runner becomes a part of it after three years. My journey in the Surf City Marathon has led me to receive many awards and many forms of recognition in many places I visit because I wear the legacy shirt and it looks excellent on me. The clubs that runners get to be in are also maintained by consistently completing marathons. If you miss a marathon in the Surf City Legacy program, then usually you need to complete three more marathons to become a part of the club again.

The Kona Brewing Company is usually the sponsor of the marathon, and since running the marathon every year since 2010, my streak is longer than most runners. The journey of running the Surf City Marathon is similar to learning how to be socially responsible and aware. By meeting a vast group of people who are leaders and others who have more personal goals, it shows a variety of individuals. Some high-profile CEOs have entered to run a marathon or half marathon and how they have a place with many other runners to finish.

In the running world and after completing a marathon, the runner can go back to their normal life and the race they ran keeps track of their finish time and information forever. Every marathon has record holders, and they know who has run the race. They often form clubs within the marathon so the runner can be a part of it. In the Orange County Marathon, there is a club called the OC Legacy Club, which is an exclusive club that runners can be a part of with rewards given to the runners each year. At the expo before the marathon, the legacy items are hot commodity with many incentives, and if you miss one year, your challenge starts over. There are many volunteers that work for the marathon who give the runners a sense of fulfillment when they pick up their items from the booth.

The race expo is usually one or two days before an event, and it just prepares you to learn about time, location, bib instructions, transportation, and what the race will bring. It is a pre-event to help the runner prepare for their race and offers free magazines, samples, advertisements, shopping, and T-shirts to runners by the race crew and event staff. Running brings many memories back because people can see and meet people that they haven't in years.

The runner goes through necessary procedures before the run to see a volunteer hand them with a prize for being in the legacy club, which leaves you with calm expression and enjoyable memories of the expo. There are people on the course that can make the run go wild. For example, in a recent OC Marathon, there were people who ride bicycles and hop into the race near the finish line during an event that get called out by the announcer, and in the LA Marathon, there are no bandits allowed in the finish line. A bandit is someone who does not wear their bib number the right way or they do not pay the fee when running in the marathon. Volunteers can even tell you to stop sleeping, and by keeping your outlook bright, you can run you race with the theme it has.

With the ten-year Beach Bum Club, there is an opportunity to get your name enshrined in a Parkers' Lighthouse bench. The location of the bench has been given by the city, and it is a way to earn some more recognition by the city of Long Beach.

Long Beach Marathon runners get to meet many people, and the course makes it a memorable experience. When you are actually on the course running, some areas are blocked off by the police, and you are in a situation where you can see a safe distance in front of you. Usually, you should run visioning ten feet ahead so you can pick up your pace if needed. It's recommended because you are keeping your eyes set on what's in front of you. Picking up your pace when needed is an important tool a runner can have because they can put more into their run at any given time. Often when running as fast as you can, you should have some precautions to prevent from collapsing, and if your body allows, you can run faster later.

In the final stretch of the Long Beach Marathon, there are sets of volunteers on the sides of the street that can give you a sense of ease as you are almost finished. They recognize your struggle to maintain a fast time for a long distance, and they see many other runners that do the same. That is when a person can see inside of themselves to feel that they are not in comparison with other runners, and soon they deserve a rest or break.

In the finish line in the Long Beach Marathon, the announcers usually call different runners' names as they finish, and once you cross the finish line, there are volunteers that hand you a medal and often congratulate you with a word of encouragement. Once you run past the finish line and go to get refreshments, some areas often serve water, bananas, or healthy food. A runner can go the challenge tent area and pick up various medals such as the California Dreamin' or

Beach Cities Challenge or other medals, depending on the race and challenges that are applicable.

Today, one of my accomplishments in running that has stood out is earning the California Dreamin' Running Award multiple times, and it's a dreamy medal. The first time I earned it was by completing the Surf City Marathon, Long Beach Marathon, and San Francisco Marathon and later earning a special medal and finisher jacket. The challenge has been discontinued, and in California, there are so many things that make the state one of the most sought after to live in. Apart from the luxurious homes, tourist spots, sports teams, and being the entertainment capital of the world, running also makes it stand out, with the Los Angeles Marathon being one of the longest running marathons. A person is said to be literally be dreaming of California when they complete the challenge because they are running in a journey through the state's landmarks. The runner is California Dreamin' because they have seen what California has to offer, and he is lucky enough have seen all the glorious landmarks and sites that the state has to offer.

A runner's sense of awareness can help them to improve their social intelligence. A runner can simply complete a challenge, or if they succumb to some of the challenges that they met along the way, they must rebound. My choice is to always run tougher and take my challenge medals with a sense of encouragement and accomplishment. It is the right choice to get your medal with a sense of pride. Often you might feel that the volunteer was expecting more from you, or you could feel that you could have communicated better with the volunteer in the short time there. Once you get past that and actually ran the race, you are able to grow. If a volunteer says, "There you go," they are usually giving you water or cheering you on. If a volunteer says, "Yep," that means that can be positive in your run because the volunteer is agreeing with you or saying yes. If I'm running and I ask for water, I later get it, which helps me stay hydrated.

My willingness to put my inspiration ahead of me and run quicker decreases the chance of pain. I often communicate more with the volunteers and often apologize and ask them to repeat something if I don't understand them or miss their message. I can take the water they gave me and focus, and it was something that I was expecting or that it's given to me now to drink. I feel that they are agreeing with me in my perceptions of my running strong and to see what's ahead of me and not get backtracked to the miscommunication earlier. Throughout the race, volunteers also help to assist me with what I need to improve.

Volunteers give me ideas of where I am with my goal of finishing, and later, I restructure my plan with keeping a constant pace so I can get to the finish line. Accomplishments take a lot of work, and many awards are given through email or mail and require applications or sending money.

Toastmasters International is headquartered in the US and is a nonprofit educational organization that works with clubs worldwide to encourage communication, pubic speaking, and leadership, and it helped me earn many awards. It creates a path to the better you. For example, I earned many Advanced Communicator Awards in my Toastmasters program and even a Distinguished Toastmasters award (DTM), which is the highest level of educational achievement with many requirements, and it made me a leader. I don't run my marathons and tell people on the course about my accomplishments, but I feel mentally prepared through my speeches, running, and coaching.

Running on hills and roads can help condition you to a faster pace, and there are opportunities to meet other runners through social media such as Facebook and Instagram and through volunteering in your community. Running safely depends on your environment, and if you enjoy social interactions, you'll find your run will be more exciting with running clubs and events. Running has led me to prepare and give many speeches that helped me to achieve my goal of a DTM, and it has showed my progress in public speaking in front of groups. I showed my medals to portray a better picture of my running experience. I feel more self-esteem and confidence while running, and the journey of my running became fun, traveling to races and increasing my pace because of consistent mileage run by me each week. I have pleasure to find safe ways through the routes of a race, and I strive to eat healthy well-balanced meals in restaurants before and after my runs.

In my work experience helping my dad at his Tax Advice Inc. business, I've seen and heard him on the phone with various Internal Revenue Service (IRS) agents to help his clients with business deals to grow their firms. The Internal Revenue Service helps people understand and meet their federal tax responsibilities, and I helped my dad mail letters to various IRS offices such as in Ogden, Utah. At the time of helping my father in his business, I didn't realize that I would actually travel to Utah for a race, and later I remembered the work I did for him. I felt a sense to enjoy my environment running the 2021 Deseret News Marathon.

My father's illness of Parkinson's disease often had my dad in the kitchen opening drawers and shelves in our home, and he had a normal mind and a business sense. He lived in various nursing homes after falling and hitting his head, causing subdural hematoma, and a broken hip bone. He was trying to be rehabilitated to walk, and he recently caught the flu or pneumonia, and he wants to walk again. He is a good person that has built life for his family and worked hard. He was first diagnosed with Parkinson's disease, Alzheimer's, and then dementia, but the feedback he's gotten from other doctors and my mom let him live in his home. He continues to seek help to feel better about himself for his family and close friends and to try to walk again. The aspect of life that has not changed from him is being himself.

Sometimes a volunteer could be so busy with so many athletes that by the time your time comes to get the medal, they seem very mindful of you and actually give more time to you. It is because you are the person who worked for the prize and achieved a medal. A runner can view a race not just for the fees to pay but also for the race to finish because they are expecting some sort of prize at the end, and once they get it, it is an upbeat experience. I run the race and feel extension of myself while running.

I listen to my heart and body enough to know that when I am pounding the pavement for 26.2 miles or more, I'm in a zone of my own. I have used my past experiences at the gym, such as at the 24 Hour Fitness reserved for indoor cycling classes and treadmill running, to get a sense of how I can motivate myself to run a marathon in around four hours. In a group exercise class at a 24 Hour Fitness, there are so many club and team members around you that make you feel comfortable to see how you've come out to a club to reap the benefits of being around other people. At work, you can run or walk to a time clock and punch in and out to perform your duties with pleasure. When trying to get a qualifying time for the Boston Marathon, you can improve your chances of qualifying by paying even more for personal training at the gym.

The reason most people take up running as a sport is to be healthier, to be more active, and to meet goals. I chose to walk with gradual steps to get leaner, and an extension of walking was to run with just a little faster hand movement. Almost every gym has treadmills to practice running, and most treadmills let the user navigate the electronics and use the technology to run, but it can be even simpler to step outside and run. The outcome of treadmill running is mostly positive because you can see and track calories burned, speed, incline, time, and heart rate.

Each time you step or run, you gain the benefits of health and social acceptance. The actual course in running is timed; and when you're at work, home, with family, friends, and coworkers, continually meeting people makes you feel better, smarter, and faster in ways. A medal earned can conglomerate your accomplishment and give you a sense of stability in your daily life.

Many treadmills can become fancier with options of routes in various places and courses such as the Eiffel Tower or a large mountain. The one thing that differs from being at the gym is that there are often fitness experts who are present with your treadmill runs, unless you have your own treadmill where you live. These fitness experts can be anything from personal trainers, to group exercise instructors, to fitness staff, or to sales people of the product.

By running on treadmills, you can prepare your body well for a run or race that is upcoming. The runner must look out for themselves to make sure that they don't overtrain and become tired before the run. Oftentimes with intense treadmill training such as seventy miles per week until a marathon, you can find yourself getting the experience of running the marathon itself. However, the course itself can differ from the training you endured because of many factors such as altitude and elevation. I've found myself that after treadmill training for various races, I had a level of confidence as far with running faster minutes per mile and running by going to group exercise classes including cycling. It gave me the extra push to see high performers, making myself feel ready to run.

Oftentimes, treadmill running can help an athlete train well for their race, but they should avoid lifting too many weights because of overtraining. Strength training and a well-balanced diet can be a way to accomplish feats in fitness and perform well, but oftentimes, overtraining can decrease performance.

In getting to a balance, I've given myself more time outside of the gym, ran more virtual and in-person runs, and worked two jobs, one as a front-end ripper, combo clerk, and courtesy clerk for Ralphs and the other as a delivery driver for Uber Eats. It helped me feel productive and less urge to overtrain. At work or in the day, you can find ways to learn to train better, and by keeping healthy boundaries with others, you can run or walk if you find space.

If I already registered and paid for a race ahead of time, it gives me a sense of joy as I run with the road ahead of me. I'm often working at Ralphs or Uber Eats, and with walking all day and communicating with customers, managers, and store employees, I can sense the race organizers have something planned that will relax me and keep me physically active. I plan for races with the help of therapy, communication with family, and people at work, and by the time I make it to the race course, I run with a positive outlook, joy, and energy. I often have other goals in mind such as Toastmasters groups, keeping a journal, and writing about my joys of running.

Relaxation and calmness are practiced in running marathons to improve areas of my life. In a work setting such as the grocery store at Ralphs, there are many light fixtures, a high ceiling, advertisements, departments, and aisles of grocery products to choose from, along with customer service at every turn. In a race that's timed, there can be various loops, turns, and aid stations to navigate, and when you finish the race on a certified course with a fast time, most of your hard work both on and off the course serves as an accomplishment to be proud of. I make the choice to smile with a customer or suggest something else to later experience a 360-degree evaluation from my colleague or supervisor and running faster and communicating smarter in real time is ongoing.

The job I have at Uber Eats as a delivery driver lets me carefully and mindfully see how business and restaurants cater to others in a way that the openness of a course brings me. By networking with different people in a customer service setting at restaurants or by greeting a host or hostess and asking for an order that was prepared for a customer, I feel the open air and an open road with beautiful scenery to view as I drive. Most races are made up by the race director and the staff who get a venue for runners to participate in. Uber Eats can be fun with one-on-one interactions with customers because by picking up food, driving, and completing an order, it enables me to better communicate when I participate and plan for a race because I feel more leisure and relaxation.

In the world of running, there is also entertainment, music, and ways to understand and process information you need to know on the course. Sometimes I question some of the things that got me to run the race, but it is temporary because when I'm on the course listening to bands play, I feel that I'm on the right track to get to the finish line. I sense that running seven- to nine-minute pace is fast enough to feel productive in the run and to finish with a faithful time. The journey today of interacting with many club team members at the local 24 Hour Fitness gym has, in a way, changed me for the better.

There are times when it is harder to exercise because of social conditions or anxieties from the day you had. In the COVID-19 pandemic, there was a shutdown of exercise facilities, but the body can still reap the benefits of the running and training that a person has done. For example, my body was still fit from the Group X classes at the 24 Hour Fitness that I participated in. There was a room in the gym for cyclists that a member could reserve classes taught by an instructor for a fee that could give you a one-on-one experience, which the fee was later not necessary because of the abundance of bikes available for the cyclists. My journey of running became interesting because of all the miles that I ran on treadmills let me feel success of my time spent.

Goals in running take time to shape, and once they are met, you can feel satisfied when you accomplish it. Currently, I look all the nearby local races that are feasible for me, and I race most of them virtually. It is pleasant to see the races that have opened back to in-person events because you have the opportunity to run in person on the course again. For a long period of time, many races have not been able to operate due to caution around the pandemic. The goals for me are often competing various running events in a series to get a certain prize or a finisher medal combing race.

In the present day, if you follow the guidelines from doctors, trainers, and physical therapists about your running properly, you can safely run with less chance of injury and head in the right direction.

In human history, my teacher from Palos Verdes Peninsula High School have talked about how viruses can potentially enter the human race and change it, such as the COVID-19 did recently. Today, with the change being seen, it made sense to me that my experience in indoor cycling made me stronger to be at an advantage in my health and exercise routine. Upon the start of the pandemic, I didn't actually believe that the world was going to end because of the shutdown of most places because of my upbringing and belief in the American system. Some people were conditioned to watch television most their lives and made some unhealthy choices in their diet and exercise, but by combining healthy choices with a healthy workout schedule or running and changing your outlook on current events, you can be an active person again.

I found that with elliptical equipment and treadmills at the local gym were pleasurable for me to keep up with my training schedule online and achieve more goals. The journey led to me to see all types of athletes such as individuals coming to exercise after work, younger kids with friends that took time off school and studying to exercise, weight lifters with capabilities to build strong muscles, or older people who just made time for themselves to get a workout in. With seeing a variety of people, it showed me that my time on the course of a marathon was well spent because I can see how the race organizers created a course with the opportunity to earn a medal.

While exercising at the gym, the experience of running can bring you 360 degrees of knowledge you gain from every action such as checking in at a gym, to changing in the locker room, to using the equipment, and to participating in classes. The experience of running on a course gives you the ability to reflect on the challenges to come out of successfully.

Since a marathon course is large and the roads are wide and blocked off for a runner, the temperature outside can be anywhere from very hot to raining. The runner is timed in the race so they are able to run at a level where they are being challenged but can also run in the fastest time. If they run accordingly at a fast pace, they can meet the challenges to give off enough power to surge ahead. The runner is able to also possibly see a difference in how their training has helped them push themselves to see positive results. In seeing the results, it can be similar to sensing that every situation you have been in now is changing to your own perception of how you should see it.

This changing of outside perceptions can last as long as you can comfortably want it to. In the gym, there are some people that can merely see you and still push you to continue your efforts to a level where you feel is necessary to have lasting change. Then there are other situations where you are just glad that you are doing the right thing for your body, but to keep your moral, you are working with the strongest athletes. The experience with running and then with breaks is usually pleasant because people are able to find a connection with the efforts they put in and the efforts they see from others. In the time of physical effort, the body can recover and be able to start a recovery that changes from the runs.

The way that the race organizers develop a clear path for the runner's finish can be similar to a trainer finding a workout for their clients. Or to put it into perspective, while exercising, you will see other trainers working with clients, which is a lot of time and effort spent on both parties. When a marathon finisher participates in running or activities at the gym, they can see that running and pushing yourself takes time. They find that when they get tired, they can see others' efforts in a way that can give a sense of relief to them.

The concept is that there are many factors that runners train for when they are in a race such as being able to keep your heart rate at a certain level. In a marathon, there are cyclists riding their bikes, musicians playing music, volunteers giving food and water, and a countless number of other things that are pleasant for the runner in their journey. In the time spent running, a runner realizes that the work they are doing is for them to show that they are capable of achievements to keep.

In marathons, a person becomes stronger with others by experience before, during, and after the race. When I exercise at the gym, I'm spending my time in a constructive manner, becoming a better person. I can use the feedback that I get during a marathon with runners that I see at the gym whether in the locker room or in another area. Greeting a club team member at the gym was an experience in its own, and I know that I'm capable to complete a lot more in my life with my goals set in the right place. I believe in myself while running and a higher power that answers some of the tougher questions to move on in my life.

Find a natural way to deal with some of the things that are more difficult such as by taking a walk or eating a fruit. Preparation for harder assignments in school can become a learning experience once you complete the assignment whether it's by essay, test, or by completing a research paper.

By August 2015, I was accepted into a business school at California State University Dominguez Hills (CSUDH) after applying to about four schools. My marathon running and experience talking in Toastmasters International groups helped me to stay on track for the eighteen months that I had in school. The changes in my schedule for running while in school caused me to exercise less, and I kept my nutrition as it was, which was not a very good level, but I worked on it. My findings of how my school related to my running were phenomenal because it was nothing but positive correlation. As I took time out of my running schedule to finish homework and study for exams, it helped me in the long run to learn how to live healthier and find ways to get past some plateaus in my training for marathons.

A similar feeling comes with running and feeling success with mental health. My mental health has always been important to me to make better decisions. By learning how to manage my money better and how to handle difficult interactions with other people, I was glad. The experience of running after setting my goals became very satisfying as I channeled my energy the right way. To try to improve my mental health so that I won't get depressed or won't relapsed to a time that was not productive is continually improving for me.

Many doctors can tell the patient that something is wrong with them, but in reality, there is nothing wrong. At this point, a runner can take whatever constructive advice they get and make it a reality. I decided to work extraordinary hours to make myself listen to suggestions and answer some of the questions that my psychiatrist had that I didn't know how to answer at one time.

In a world of resources, a runner has a variety of ways to improve their running such as meeting various people that they wouldn't normally meet and communication about safe ways to meet their goals. My quest in marathon running has brought me to a number of paths to improve my pace, which has improved with more preparation and running every day. My pace also improves through productivity in the working world, treadmill running, and running in my neighborhood because my body is functioning and exerting energy. The way to feel your mood enhance is by seeing the various people on the course and view it as an ongoing learning experience because most runners want to have fun. When I was in graduate school at CSUDH, I learned various business theories and applied them in class or other places, which showed me that my time was spent constructively.

Besides the Long Beach Marathon, the other race that I have run consciously for at least ten years was the Los Angeles Marathon. The Los Angeles Marathon awarded me with a ten-year medal. The experience for me was exciting because by being loyal to the LA Marathon for ten years, they finally recognized me with a special medal. There was one year in 2010 that I volunteered for the LA

Marathon, and it was a major change from running because I felt more stationary because of not running.

Volunteering for the 2010 LA Marathon was a unique experience because it was the first time I decided to volunteer for the race. A customer and reporter at one of my previous places of employment called the MHA Village to ask me if I was going to run the LA Marathon that year. I usually run the race every year, but at that time, I had feelings about work that often had me feel lazy. At that time, I wasn't fully motivated to participate in outside events, and I decided to volunteer because I did not sign up as a runner in time.

Upon arriving to the LA Marathon in 2010, there were a few aid stations where I assisted giving water to the runners. In one station, I offered refreshments to runners, and I felt a sense of boredom because I was used to being in the fast lane running, and that's where I decided to be from there.

The Los Angeles Marathon has a lot of hills, and the course changes often and sometimes takes longer for some to finish than others. Running through the hills is usually pleasant, and having volunteers on your side while running that give you praise helps push me through each race. The idea that I can beat my personal record (PR) in any race helps me to stay driven after each race.

Recently with an app called Runkeeper, I improved my PR in many categories such as most calories burned in a week, most hills climbed in a week, and most floors climbed in a week. I conquered a lot of these goals and achieved the feet through being able to adjust to a work schedule with my previous job at Elite Development Enterprises as an account manager. There were days where I go to the office by 8:30 a.m. or 10:30 a.m. and left by 11:00 a.m. to go to the field, which is actual neighborhoods, and present sales of attic insulation.

In my job as an account manager at Elite Development Enterprises, I had the pleasure of informing customers about LADWP's attic insulation rebate program, and I had a sales pitch that was practiced with my team every morning and evening. The morning hours at that job consisted of an AM ATMO where I would practice my sales pitch with coworkers and improve my confidence and selling ability with others. After eating lunch, I would drive to the field where I would walk for nearly seven hours a day, greet and meet customers in residential areas, which proves to be a new training ground.

Oftentimes in the starting line for a race, there are a large number of random people warming up for the race and meeting each other. The purpose is to feel comfortable with other runners and to make new friends, push yourself to run faster, and have pleasant motivation throughout the race.

When meeting customers and explaining how they could benefit from attic insulation in the company I worked called Superhero, it showed that I was breaking grounds to learn how to communicate well enough to make a customer feel like they can welcome me in their home and enjoy the benefits of the product I showed them.

At Elite Development Enterprises, my duties of working in the field were similar to how a police officer or detective goes to work to make money. My duties were going door-to-door and help to inform customers for opportunities to insulate their attic. It was a path proven to be successful for many account managers to eventually own their own office and become a business owner. A job earning minimum wage can be an option for people who do not want to work as many as ninety hours per week.

The idea of selling products to customers can create a life for you or you can earn a living. By assisting people with various products and later running, you can find yourself keeping a marathoner's pace. For example, the sales process of attic insulation can be a way to motivate yourself to go out for a run. The pace that is set by those who sell products also needs to be matched by others in the business to measure up. If a story is told at work about a couple of people who have really made a name for themselves by performing well in sales, they can be an example of how others can do the same. When a winner of a marathon talks to the press or media about their journey or how they got there, they, too, can be an example of how other runners can do the same. Many runners are sponsored by a clothing or shoe brand, or they also have companies themselves to run.

While being out in the field, I knocked on hundreds of doors every week and created a sense of confidence in my running style that helped me train at a special level. The hours of walking and communicating with people gave me habits and a sense of confidence in my daily routine. With the time I spent at home with my father and knowing my mother had experience working with people who were patients as a nurse, my sense of purpose at home was welcoming. The effects that running has on a person's mental attitude can show when you are working to help with triumph.

The sayings "Too much is never enough" and "You only have one cup of energy left in you" are ones that I appreciate. The fact that my ability to have time to reap the benefits of my running is one that I have gratitude for. After finishing various running events, there are finish line events and ways volunteers who help with massages that make a lasting change on the event.

The changes for me from training at the local 24 Hour Fitness for eight hours a day to walking through neighborhoods in Los Angeles, Venice, San Pedro, Wilmington, and South LA was the actual time spent in the gym to being outside. My actual time of using the treadmills, weight sets, cardiovascular equipment, and being in the facility dropped from eight hours to nearly two hours with the usual four visits a day. The only difference was that instead of going to a local super sport gym in Torrance/PV, I went to the Downtown Long Beach Super Sport gym.

I knew that I was spending my time the right way with my physical activity and training for my marathons because I saw the various team members and trainers working with the other members too. Today, Elite Development Enterprises has closed, and the walking I learned has stayed with me.

There can be roadblocks to go from a sedentary lifestyle to an elite athlete. Once you get to the position of an athlete, you can think and act differently from where you were or you can progress as a person and eat proper meals. If you missed a workout because you had no time, it is in your lifestyle to maintain a lean body. My work schedule was irregular, and since I had prestige and a steady school schedule when earning my master of business administration degree in California State University Dominguez Hills, it became a goal to succeed through Elite Development Enterprises company's eight- to twelve-month management training program at one time. In an ultramarathon, you must accept and follow through the course without doubt.

The experience I had in my ultramarathon in San Francisco makes the hours at work seem as a piece of cake. Why would I worry about my hours spent at work when I already have an ultramarathon under my belt? If I see others competing to outperform, there has to be something that gives, and something gave—my sleep.

At my previous position as an account manager, the day started one hour and a half later because of management's decision to experiment with it while monitoring productivity. The guidelines with the coronavirus have the office closed temporarily and today permanently because of the Centers for Disease Control and Prevention's guidelines. While I was selling attic insulation door-to-door or working as a delivery driver, I was using my time to work and later achieved more in my runs.

My transition from the long hours of exercise to the long hours of work can serve as an example to help runners realize that in their journey, they have potential for upward progression. The joy of running can enlighten your life with faster runs. In my recent in-person LaceUp Ventura Marathon, which was one run in a series of four runs called the LaceUp Running Series, I achieved my fastest time in a marathon, at about 3:39. There were three other cities in addition to Ventura for the LaceUp Running Series: Palos Verdes, Riverside, and Orange County.

No matter how much time you prepare for an event, there is something that you'll probably forget before the start of the race, but do not let that stop you! Whether it is forgetting to turn your door light off in your car, forgetting a pair of shoes in another location, forgetting a certain medication prescription, or not bringing a charger, there are things that you'll forget, but try to take it as a learning experience and grow stronger from it and have more experiences for your next run.

The LaceUp Running Series was a series that was considered one of the best running courses because of the scenic areas. It was a combination of full and half marathons and included a challenge medal after finishing four races in one year. The Palos Verdes Half Marathon was close to where I live. I registered for it, and the course was familiar because I ran nearby Palos Verdes Marathon the last year it was scheduled, which was in 2011. Palos Verdes was runner up to the Boston Marathon for the best courses in the United States of America, but it was discontinued perhaps because of the location being so stunning. The LaceUp Running Series was recently canceled, and it had four races that worked with Series Runner, including Riverside, Palos Verdes, Orange County, and the Ventura Marathon, and I felt bright to earn a four-race challenge medal at the last race with Series Runner in the series that year.

By having self-assurance in your training plan, you are better off than most other runners because you have found some sort of autonomy or well-being in your training. Whether you have improved your PR from your last race or you have learned how to run a race without asking as many questions as you once did, you can show yourself that you have improved your ability and poise to run fast. By looking at my workout history online for my past month or two, I can see the effort I put into getting out in the world of fitness to improve how I interact with people and athletes who train smarter.

Control with time and focus in a race is essential, and you can communicate with others before the start of the marathon. Run under control well enough in the first half so you know you have energy for the second half. Most of the time, you can sense your energy level during the first half of race and run at a pace that is more comfortable for you to finish. There is the saying that you only have one cup of energy left, which means that no matter how hard you train and run, you only have one cup of coffee or you're as good as the last sip. My decision to stop drinking coffee with caffeine has also helped me to maintain more natural energy and avoid exhaustion before sleep. By cutting out caffeine in my diet from everything from Clif shots to green tea, my natural level of energy has raised.

Collection in running means that your thought remains objective so you are not distracted during a run. A collection of medals or harder-sought medals can be gratifying to you at any time. Some forms of distraction to look out for that can cause you to lose time in marathons are spectators outside of the course sidelines, but it is important that your attention is not on them and instead on yourself. A way to avoid spectators' distractions is to not make eye contact with the large crowds of people that you do not know.

The strategy to focus on yourself and keep your goal of finishing strong can bring you a sense of inspiration. A little-known fact about marathons is that there is a finish line and keep in mind you are bound to get there. The race is composed of 26.2 miles formed by a race director and others so that after the race, you can rest, recollect your thoughts, and go back to your normal life with added coolness. It is ensuring to know you can trust a race to put on an event that you'll enjoy.

There are more ways to train smarter in the gym such as personal training that can also improve your marathon time, but it might seem unreasonable because of the costs. With the choice to use all your resources, you might find yourself looking at some things that you could have done instead of taking the time to train more. For instance, after looking at a web page that shows training packages a gym offers with more fees, it can seem extreme. It is similar to jumping hurdles. Once you jump past one, there is another and another until you complete the set and can say for yourself that your run is done. Oftentimes, being able to work and earn income can be a better choice.

In the corporate world, many executives start from the bottom and work their way up the ladder to advance in their careers. In running, many can start as being disabled and work their way to feel they are no longer disabled and competent to take on the tasks of the real world in real time. The way to run on a course, learn from it, leave some ideas aside, and be comfortable is vital in life.

For example, Intel had a CEO who ran a half marathon, and it made a story in *Bloomberg Businessweek* magazine. It shows you that the work you do for a marathon is noted well for you and by others.

The stigma that people have about some things vanishes in races because you are able to see how a course is set the same for everyone. You can broaden your outlook to learn more about how to be wiser in your thinking if you encounter more difficult parts to lessen life's pressures as they arise.

After quitting drinking alcohol, my experience with the Surf City Marathon and others has developed. Most people gear up with food and drinks before Superbowl Sunday and support a common theme of family and let loose and have fun. By running in the marathon, a lot of memories arise as to when I used to do something to fit in better and how it makes me feel now. There is motivation that a runner builds up throughout their free time by interacting better with others. Various training plans are needed because by the time you see some volunteers on the sidelines either giving you water, motivating you, or cleaning the area up, your physical effort is at a very high level and you can make it a positive experience. The unique part of running is that with whatever level of training you do, either at the gym or running outside, you'll find a way to appreciate your own hard work and not have any feelings of doubt.

There are many ways runners can gear up for a marathon, such as by using a Runkeeper app, which puts the run-on calendar for you in preparation for your run. A safe way is to gear up is to run your miles that are scheduled, have the running gear you need, and drink plenty of liquids and healthy food. Your running can make you enjoy food more, have a better appetite, and live with energy and happiness. The running journey is a balance of mental and physical goals to meet, and the effort in a run brings positive reactions by others.

It is a euphoric feeling running on your own with a fast pace, and the energy that was exerted can go toward your next experiences. Something that has helped me in my athletic training is being able to weigh myself once every two days instead of daily. With my state-of-the-art Fitbit Aria 2 scale and now the Aria Air scale, there is a setting for athletic people such as marathon runners that helps me track goals and progress. The technology in the world today lets a person reap the benefits in many ways.

While running in a straight path and hearing yourself with the crowd, you can find a level of comfort that is special, and it lets you continue to run as fast as you can to the finish line. Sometimes you make yourself ask, what is it that made you run faster? What is it that motivated you? Can you still have this motivation at other times when you need it?

Oftentimes, the preparation that a runner does to improve themselves can help in the short term and long term to run with more sureness. The proof is in how you feel during the run and finding it again and again that can help you as a runner. The series of steps and movements that it takes to get in rhythm are important to feel you're running well. Perhaps you can sprint three miles at time without fatigue, but instead, you are experiencing yourself wanting to push harder when it is hard. The way to handle the outside crowd while running is to keep your sense of effort and willpower within you long enough to not be distracted. While running a longer distance, the journey can seem to be more of a test to see how your spirit can interplay with your sense of how the people are cheering.

My interactions either at home, driving, going to the gym, going to work, or greeting family or guests during the regular season or holiday season has myself feel ready for a run. During the run itself, my body often takes a different route that seems to run faster past different gas stations and places of business that are there, but as the runner, the time is on my side. Holidays can be unique situations and many races wish you happy holidays, and while I'm running, I show gratitude and patience toward my family, coworkers, friends, and the community while running. When the holidays come such as Fourth of July, they are enjoyed in a unique way because of the day off, and some marathons choose to have events on holidays, and others are enjoyed at certain times of the year.

The difference between an ultramarathon and a marathon is enormous. The change in events was not too much to grasp at first because I was used to volunteers lining up to help and aid runners such as myself to perform well. The main difference in the volunteers was that I noticed more time spent in preparing for the marathon than those who helped in the ultramarathon. By the time twenty-one miles came in the first lap of the ultramarathon, I saw a volunteer and asked her if she had water; her response to me was that "Hmm, would you like a peanut butter and jelly sandwich?" Later, I felt very satisfied to take it, and the struggles of finding a suitable toilet and right path in the run were later solved.

Time off in running is a way for others to catch up in their occupation. In the running world at the expo of a marathon, there are a group of vendors who have professional experience in selling products that see you to purchase their product and make you feel on track. There are various people with you who understand your effort with the vendors. The big marathon events such as the San Francisco Marathon and Ultramarathon can make you feel a high purpose of being at the event as they agree or relate with you in conversation in your journey of preparation before the race itself. As an encouragement, try to continue to do what makes you feel effective in your running and share your knowledge with others because there are volunteers who are working to help you in your race.

The body does not want to over exhaust itself when training to make yourself uncomfortable in your abilities to perform well when you run the race. A learning opportunity is that while you're on the course running, the event you are in is a different place than before, and you can picture or envision yourself to perform better now. For example, in my ultramarathon in San Francisco, I got to a point in the course near the end of the first marathon where I saw various people operating machinery in the docks, and some random people came up to me and said it was okay.

At my 2019 San Francisco Ultramarathon, I mostly saw people in the streets gathering together along with some without homes, who often offered encouraging things to say while some didn't. I felt togetherness with my fellow runners to conversate about anything for inspiration. At first, I needed to push a little bit harder because as a human myself, I can sense the various levels of challenges that I must get through while running in addition to the words of encouragement or feelings I have for myself while running.

In my second ultramarathon in San Francisco, there were four aid stops, and each one was a positive experience because of the communication and the snacks. It was thrilling to be running on pace at about eight minutes per mile in the start to about twelve minutes per mile later. My emotions were stable, and with the snacks, the volunteers were friendly enough to talk to me about my progress and took note of my number. I felt as if I were on a roll by my fellow runners asking me my secrets when I told them that I wanted to keep the goal of the first lap in mind while eating healthy and looking forward to the second lap.

The experience in the ultramarathon guided me to learn how to run faster and cleverer. Since there were only about seventy runners in the race, it felt fine to talk to one another to find the right route in the course. The assistance from the race directors and the staff during the race was helpful for me to have an understanding in accordance to where I needed to go. After finishing my first lap or marathon in the ultramarathon, I visited the event staff and was congratulated for finishing the first lap. My ability to change and get ready for the next lap was done well because of my excitement toward the other runners. My body felt fine, and I knew the reactions that I'd get would be a little mixed because most people would be tired.

There were some volunteers who also handed out energy drinks before the second lap. Since I brought my own nutrition to the run, I did not need to rely so much on the extra things that the volunteers had to drink or eat. By asking the right questions to the right people, I was in a boat that was going the right direction.

Perhaps instead of bringing a certain number of protein bars, which was often thirty-five protein bars, I could have brought sixteen or six, and today I wouldn't bring any. It was in an email chat with my Runcoach training program that a coach told me that they would never recommend bringing thirty-five protein bars to a run. The protein bars didn't help me too much, and often I would save the rest for a later time. At the ultramarathon, I kept half of my bars in the Hyatt hotel before the actual second half of the race. It helped me carry less in the first half of the run.

When asking a question to a training program, you should try get as many viewpoints as possible with the answer. Today, I simply trust the race organizers enough with the course nutrition they offer unless it has caffeine, and I don't feel it's necessary anymore to bring my own protein bars unless I'm hungry before the race. Oftentimes, the whey protein in milk and in the protein bars can make my stomach upset. There can be a social pressure in saving protein bars until after the race because you should enjoy everything you have with you on the course and later enjoy the finish line refreshments more.

The training programs that I use today are rather expensive for the average person, and I also could have more programs that help me, but by saving money when needed, it helps to keep me ready for a race.

The big picture of running an ultramarathon in San Francisco is to see where you are and where you are going for your run. In a city that is famous for the Golden Gate Bridge, an idea that intrigues me is that since the bridge is on the back of most California State drivers' licenses or IDs, it says something about the state of California itself of how people enjoy free time and are able to live their day-to-day lives with purpose. By having a vision of where I am now, I can also have a vision of how I will be running and pushing my body in another time in the future. Even though humans cannot go into the future, they can have a better future with the work they put in today.

My journey of finishing the second lap of the San Francisco Ultramarathon was similar to other marathons that I've completed in San Francisco. However, the only difference was that I was a little more tired before the run. In my efforts in the run, there was a time when I needed to walk a little bit of the course because my muscles were a little cramped. After picking myself up from walking, I noticed the volunteers were very excited to give me water, but they also moved themselves to a point that they made me work harder. People often differentiate how they react to me if they do not know me, and some interact with me as if they did. I'm able to interact with people that I have not met, and life is more meaningful because I can build relationships with people and I can help them.

In marathon running, there is always more to learn, and the human body can still push farther for you to get a more complete picture of yourself and how you see the world. For example, after my first San Francisco Ultramarathon, I heard of a website called

UltraSignup, which has various smaller distance runs to larger runs. Some of the ultramarathons are one hundred miles or more, which are for the most experienced runners. Often, qualifications to make it to an ultramarathon are to run a fifty-mile run and also a one hundred-mile run.

A runner's pace can be improved in a variety of ways, and one is to time yourself for a mile and run through another mile to beat your time. You can time yourself by walking the dog, taking a walk at work, running outside your home, or running normal tasks and errands at home and see the average change. By taking the average time of a mile, my pace is anywhere from five minutes to thirty minutes. Pace can also be improved by listening to the various coaching strategies from successful renowned coaches as you pass others. Finding races to run and qualify for and completing special challenges are interesting to find.

In finding ways to train better, try to find out what you excel in and use it to your advantage. For example, by finding the types of exercises you are better at such as treadmill running and some you could improve on such as running outside, you can learn to take breaks after a number of miles to hydrate for your body to adapt. Before a race, my intentions were to be prepared on the course and run from start to finish at a constant pace. After the race, I could relax, take in the air, enjoy myself and the atmosphere around me, and feel that another race was completed. Having the ability to communicate with others without sitting down and stopping can uplift your spirit, and you can take the time to walk for fifteen minutes after the race to stay active.

In the world of exercise, although running on the treadmill is important, running outside in the environment lets the body experiences more, can be better for your joints, and is less expensive. By watching the news on television, the headlines are perceived, but the careful thing to do is not to be overly influenced by news stories and to feel that your own run lets you perceive the outside world better. Many people in the running world have running clubs or training programs that help them maintain a fixed schedule with miles run per week or month. The clubs can be an excellent tool to find ways to run faster that cost money, but if you are running daily, you can log your miles with an online training program or by yourself.

As long as you have some kind of adequate training schedule with running, working out, or walking, you are able to use coaches to your advantage. If you start to set aside time and money toward improving your running, you can successfully see your results improve with your runs. In my experience, oftentimes I was spending too much time and money on my running apps and exercise that my training could often be overdone. By many attempts to give and take with my training whether by sleeping more or exercising less, working more, and studying more, I've found balance that helps me feel stronger in my running efforts.

Runcoach, Strava, Runkeeper, Future, and the Nike app are training programs that I participate with that give me a certain number of miles to run weekly for races that give medals. By walking at my job at Ralphs as a combo clerk and with Uber Eats as a delivery driver, I'm walking the equivalent distance of miles that are assigned to run, and often I log them. The Runcoach training program allows me to chat with the coaches about any questions, and they give me high fives as recognition for completing a run.

The training regimen the Future app by 24 Hour Fitness often had me run or walk ten miles a day, two days per week, or four workouts per week to complete. The app gives me feedback from the coach, and I often shorten the runs and get guidance with healthy eating and the proper way to train and recover. I often ran a marathon in a day, and two or three half marathons in the same week, which made me optimistic to get two to three days' rest. The races I ran with the app try to give me a different opportunity to race safely while still managing other parts of my life well.

The interesting part of running is that by the time you get to the starting line of a race or marathon, you will see that there are many other runners with you and different in respect to how they've trained. A word of wisdom is to try to notice and continue the practices that are comforting in life and continue them. Find the items that make life easier for you whether it is writing in a journal, reading a book, conversing with family, or any other hobby that excites you, and be yourself. Live the journey so you can handle the surprises that life throws at you cooler.

Feeling your accomplishments in life is another path that takes time and effort to sustain because you should give yourself a treat when you succeed. It is easy for someone who is in a different position than you are and that does not know too much about you to affect your own viewpoint of an accomplishment. Many employers have a way of formally recognizing their employees for their hard work and accomplishments such as by giving them a bonus or a certificate. In a place such as a gym, you often build yourself up as a person with confidence by having goals and knowing a way to get there. By finishing an ultramarathon, you can carry your confidence to have bragging rights because you have completed the event.

The way to find balance, a positive attitude, and live your life with the edge is the reason that many people start running. The accomplishment of an ultramarathon can help someone get through brain surgery because the neurosurgeon's job does not seem to be difficult, given the runner's efforts that brought them there. A runner can go through a journey while attending the expo for an event, and it is often said not to attend the race expo for more than one hour. Too much time at an expo isn't worthwhile to a runner because most importantly he has to focus his energy on running the race the next day or two.

In a race expo, there are many vendors that assist the runners with everything, from purchasing T-shirts to winning vacation in Hawaii. In the expo, the vendors usually provide samples of various drinks or food, and they have exhibits with different professionals in their field that provide anything from free chiropractic exams to stretching clinics.

My journey of running lets me take a bigger look into the profession to see where I place in the sport and society as a whole. For example, there are many business professions available, and since I studied general business as a major on campus for my MBA from CSUDH, I'm very knowledgeable in the field of business as a whole. When I look at how other fields such as medicine or law give the person a place to practice such as a doctor's office or courthouse, I see how someone prepares to use it every day. Running is a sport that does not really require an office, and people look at runners more as athletes that enjoy the sport. The professionals in different fields who run as a sport are no longer in the office, and they can run for a medal, which makes the sport enjoyable and exhilarating for the ones who put forth more effort.

The running journey starts with you, and at every instant, there are commercials on television, programming, news articles, and informercials that grasp your attention and make you lazy. By reading through stories and understanding various topics, you learn to relate your own ideas to others better. When a person reads the front page of the newspaper, they know what's going on in the world, which is important. It can help you have an idea or to create a blueprint for the day, and it's up to you on how to apply it to flourish. In the running community, there are many blogs and pieces of information to read in magazines or websites that help runners from anything such as how to stretch better in between runs to having proper form when they run.

The feeling that comes with running in a marathon in a different town, city, or state can be a waking point for me because I can use my two feet to explore the city and enjoy my surroundings. In most marathons, the name often comes from the city where the race is located. For example, the SDDCU Orange County (OC) Marathon is located in Orange County or Costa Mesa, California, and starts at the Newport Beach Marriott Hotel and Spa ang goes through attractive shoreline communities of Newport Beach, Costa Mesa, and Santa Ana and finishes at the OC Fair and Event Center. I go through the cities with the runners in manner of casually viewing the nice houses and views in the area similar to someone being treated by a tour guide.

An exciting feature of participating in groups is getting to talk about my future runs and runs that I've completed. The experience of the meeting that a runner gets is to meet new people and starts to appreciate life similar to when people start a new job; they see different kinds of people.

The Orange County Marathon also supports Kids Run the OC, which is a KROC training program that educates kids how to be active and have healthy lifestyles to battle childhood overweight and improve overall well-being. The goal is "inspiring kids to fitness" through fun, collaborative games and challenges. When I run the OC Marathon, the kids run their own event, and oftentimes I see kids that run the longer distance races by themselves or with family, which can make me feel as though I'm helping the kids run.

The Orange County Marathon has an excellent reputation for its course and scenery. The aspect that sets it apart from others is that along the course, you'll see various police cadet volunteers that are younger in age who seem to help you through the course. They keep the course somewhat exciting because they are able to look at the runners and communicate with each other about various topics of interest and safety. It could be that the cadets are representing how much preparation a runner feels that they have committed during a run or just making them feel safe.

The journey of running also leads a person to recovery because after you finish your run, you can find time to recover your muscles and stretch your body. For example, in the Orange County Marathon, there is a place for runners to get a massage after the run called Massage Envy. My experience is that after running the 26.2-mile race and after I pass through the finisher's area and get refreshments such as Gatorade, protein bars, or other snacks, I feel that the race has changed my outlook on life for the better with no strings attached. When I make my way to the massage tent, there are staff members taking information from the runners with clipboards for a free massage, and by being there, I can recoup.

A light in the end of the tunnel is usually the finish line, which is the primary motivation for a runner, and when it comes the time to relax after a race, their massage areas have volunteers that answer your questions. The wait in line for a massage after a marathon has many runners telling different stories from their running. Before and after the race, there are many volunteers who socialize with other runners to help them race with confidence.

For example, recently in line for a massage after an OC Marathon, I started to chat with many runners about my time achieved for the race, how many marathons I've run to date, and how many challenges I've completed. Also where I am in the current challenge series of the race, which marathons I've run, which marathons are my favorite, how often I train, how I try to avoid injury, and some of my likes and dislikes as a person. Later, I ask the runner about themselves too and about their experience with the run, their favorite run, how they train, how often they train, and also about whether or not they are going to run another marathon, which make remarkable stories to remember.

The journey of meeting different people in marathons builds ways for you to keep healthy relationships. There have been times that I feel like I'm going around in circles with similar feedback either in group therapy where I can get drowsy because of the lack of interest. My lifestyle differs because of exercise and training, and in the brief recovery time after a marathon, I meet similar people with names on their bibs, and I break the ice and meet them and learn about them well enough to feel adequate in my running expedition.

Marathons are set up by the race director as fine-tuned and designed well enough so after the runner is finished with the race, they can say their time was spent well and positively enough to enjoy their glorious moment. In the OC Marathon, there is also an area in the finish line to have a slice of pizza, but my choice was to take off the cheese and enjoy the food the way it was without guilt.

The finish line party of the Orange County Marathon was structured well with bands playing live music, runners cheering, dancing, and vendors in booths either selling merchandise at a discounted price or giving away free energy drinks. The atmosphere after a marathon often is calm; most runners are prepared to leave the race right after the event, and some runners prefer to enjoy the festivities with friends and family.

The journey after a marathon can be relaxing because you are in control of your surroundings just as you were running each mile, but now as you settle into your body and go about your day, you are approaching your day or night with newfound strength, confidence, and joy. I find ways to channel my energy into reading, meeting people, talking with family, eating healthy meals, understanding television shows better, and also updating my training logs with my race results.

After passing the finish line, you need to follow safety guidelines to go home. A runner could typically spend hours after the finish line of a race either by waiting in line for a massage, hanging out in the beer garden, going to a finish line party, or waiting in the family reunion area for family, which is because you have the freedom to spend time as you want to. After finishing the race, there are runners behind you and in front of you. One time, my Fitbit Flyers, which are music headphones compatible for my Fitbit Ionic, must have been misplaced in the massage area after a recent Surf City Marathon Event, and they weren't found. I checked the lost and found for my Flyers, and I asked many volunteers of the race if they found them, but there was no luck.

When seeing the runners past the finish line, I still felt a sense of honor in being able to feel a little bit faster than others, and they seemed to enjoy the event. There is a way to wear your headphones so that they do not get lost; just do not let people see them. The more you apply what you've learned on the course for the next race, the better chances you have to an improved run.

The competition in running can be used to help the runner have a healthy vision of where they are and where they want to be. The more a runner uses their resources such as the apps on their phone, the more the runner feels they have a well-guided race ahead of them. Oftentimes, a race has SMS texts for results to be viewed instantly. A healthy way to view competition is to let the other runners help you run faster as you continue to focus on yourself and your running capabilities.

Often the change a person makes from getting out of bed, putting their running shoes on, and leaving the home to run can make a person feel tired and not run as hard. The tool that helps me is to breathe through my nose when running and to try to use my mouth in breathing out to make the extra pushes toward a faster running time.

When I run, I feel like my lungs take in the air. I practice breathing techniques to run healthier. Many social situations that lead up to the race such as shopping, new events, and socializing have changed my attitude for the better. My drive to work and accomplish goals in running has advanced because I stopped comparing myself and I'm careful not to overstep and disrespect another person. Many runners find ways to run faster in their own way, and I carefully communicate throughout the day and take the steps toward believing more in myself and others do too.

There are many platforms where a runner can check their results online, and usually after a race, there are computers where you can view your results by name or with your iPhone. There is one website called RunRaceResults, which lists the previous years' races in a tab and also gives the runner the option to view their finisher certificate online. The results are loaded after the participant enters their first and last name with bib number, and the race filters are seen with their name with the race organization logo side by side. A runner can feel healthy competition or a competitive nature during a race by being mindful when making eye contact with participants of the race.

The journey of running a marathon provides instances where you can improve your form by seeing how other runners' bodies move as they run. By searching for your race online or by signing up for an email list for a race, it balances your physical health with emotional health and save yourself the time and energy. By improving your emotional health and enjoying your runs, you can be more content with running because you'll experience more and feel better. Being able to motivate yourself in more ways than one is important for runners to get an extra push.

There is a lot of motivation used for each run I race, which is mainly used through long distance running, and the changes are felt crossing the street at a crosswalk or when my route changes due to the hills. A runner needs to have self-awareness as to how their feels through proper self-preparation techniques such as stretching before a run. The more a runner stretches their muscles, the more conditioned they will be when their body feels like cramping or giving up.

The more techniques that you use to stretch, the better you'll recover your body when you cramp or feel it's difficult during a run. A proper diet plan shows that the food you put into your body makes you feel the same way or, as the saying goes, junk in, junk out. A donut or cheeseburger usually has harsh effects on your arteries because the saturated fat is much harder to burn than foods with polyunsaturated fat such as avocado.

Every runner should have a journey to tell that shows steps that others can follow for achievement. The steps for a leaner and stronger body often come with proper diet, exercise, training, discipline, motivation, practice, and persistence. The select few that often win the race have done so through running on coals in their homeland or running as a ritual practice with a lifestyle that matches their countries' culture. In Ethiopia, there are runners that live a close culture with their family to run seventy miles a week while they put forth effort when they do daily chores such as wash their clothes and converse with family.

In 2018, I had the opportunity to train with Beit T'Shuvah, which is a residential addiction treatment center that trains for the Los Angeles Marathon. The night before the marathon, we were brought to a hotel that was rented that had a carb-loaded dinner. Some of the fastest sponsored runners from Africa entered the hotel building and seemed interested that we put forth an effort to train together before the marathon.

The training that comes before a marathon can either make the runner ready in an instant or make the runner feel as though they put a lot of time in one area of training while they could have focused on other ways. The comradery and feelings of hard work can last to the starting line. My ability to greet some of the runners that were on my team before the race were followed by a thirty-minute delay. While running the race, I saw the person that I stayed with in my hotel the night before, and he joked with me as to how well we were and that the porta potty line was short.

This is a beautiful aspect in running to shine because you are exerting yourself with your hard work with many people around, and you feel as though your experience two hours ago has passed. It is similar to when two people have a conversation, there is a time when there are bumps in the conversation because you are trying to either dispute something or agree about something, but when you get the hindsight about what was said, you make ends meet.

Many online training programs have often professional coaches that guide you to success. Some online programs help a runner twenty-four hours a day, seven days a week. Runcoach is one of the programs that a runner can use where the coaches give you high fives after your race is completed. High fives are special because you've shown another person that you passed a time of your life that required hard work. It is a confirmation online with coaches to acknowledge your achievement.

A high five also can be exciting when you are finishing a marathon as you notice other runners with the work they do. Running brings about a lot of smiles as the human body gets to another level and form with you as the driver. Sports such as bodybuilding, tennis, football, basketball, baseball, and golf have the body move and travel to let the athlete feel well and fine-tuned. The body turns in a motion and functions with various forms with running. Professional athletes in each of these sports put forth a lot of physical effort and energy, and their body works well with the mind when finishing a marathon.

The journey of continually perceiving various stimuli in the mind and making sense of it can give you a sense of enthusiasm to discover more about yourself. When I practice running or walking either by training on my own or working at various jobs, there is an absorbing experience.

Most runners train to the level of skill they have, and a professional runner might run about fifteen to seventeen miles around their home daily, consistently eating healthy meals and snacks, and a have social lifestyle at home with loved ones. Instead of running eighteen miles outside of my home or on trails, I would go for a run on pavement outside. I've found that exercise on treadmills at the local gym with a number of miles works too.

When a running event comes closer such as a marathon or ultramarathon, the community or society prepares for it, and there's enough time to train for the event. The reason could be that the event has many sponsors that help running the community or it's filled with so many people that the city takes time to prepare the roads for race and often lets the runners know which roads will be closed.

There is more time to train and be with family near the holidays, and there have been some unforeseen events to alter the way you train. In the recent coronavirus pandemic, there was a situation where most people left their offices at work to meet the community's guidelines to be home all day. That left me more time to train for the ultramarathon in San Francisco. At one time, I was working nearly three hundred hours for months, and I felt that it would continue and that I couldn't continue the regular running training that I was used to.

In my recent memories for the ultramarathon, the course was very beautiful and the areas through San Francisco were amazing to see now that I can train by running more miles before a race.

The training level differs for each type of competitor in a race, and with all the training that a runner completes, he can see all the effort in their results with each race, mile after mile. I usually have some form of consistent training either at the gym with classes, at home, at work, or by eating healthy, which can bring my time in a marathon to four hours and thirty minutes or better. If I run more outdoors or a eat a better-balanced meal, my lifestyle adjusts from spending hours at the gym to running more on my own. By working more consistent hours at work, there could be a change for the better. In the first few miles of the race, I can see the different runners who start in the first wave to be together. While in my run, my focus changes to the runners ahead and to the volunteers on the sidelines giving water or refreshments. The change of considering how the sidelines is situated with more volunteers can be good because I know that my effort is given.

The journey of finding the right training technique always changes, and as much as a person train for a run, they always find ways to enhance their talents. The training for a run can also be expensive because there are people who will see you that you need to change or improve something. The way some people can take charge and feel confident in themselves that they have done enough is a trait that more people should have.

Today, it is often unknown to know where your classmates have gone and where they stand physically and socially when some might not still be around or have moved on. For example, when I was a senior in high school, after graduating from Palos Verdes Peninsula High School, there was something called a grad night where the roles seemed to change because there was a fun night planned. I saw older people in groups who were not educators on campus playing various games with us as students and giving us okays in many of the social situations that were fun for us as classmates. Oftentimes when running a marathon, there are so many people you don't really know cheering you on for your effort, either volunteers or supporters, that let you experience many constructive emotions.

As a person enters college, there are many changes in the way the educators help the students and the way the student plans for life activities after graduation. The student can graduate and become an alumnus of the university, and they are given the decision to go to graduate school and become as double alumnus of CSUDH. It let me experience different alumni events such as a dodger baseball game where I got to sit near other alumni that had different experiences after college than mine or by going kayaking in Long Beach and playing beach games. I still stay in touch with many people after my graduation, and I excel in many areas of my life.

Feedback from the outside world, volunteers, spectators, and runners can improve your training regimen. Running outside my home and seeing the environment often gives me a runny nose, and I now bring tissues with me. Some of the hills become less challenging with experience, and my pace can also improve through listening to feedback. If something makes me ponder, it is usually a positive thing because the people who are around me are either working or communicating about some part of their day, where someone is in their day differs from person to person. Some feedback has allowed me to participate more in various challenges to use my full effort, and my end goal of becoming more at peace with myself matters most.

A few things to consider in your running journey is where you are and what time it is. Whether it is Monday, Tuesday, Wednesday, Thursday, Friday, Saturday, or Sunday or 7:00 a.m., 7:00 p.m., or any other time, there are people that you communicate with to share similar perceptions for events and ideas. The weekends are the time that people usually have more time to relax and not work, where they interact more with people at the local store or restaurant about how their week was.

The start of the week is often on Monday, and there's a social aspect that's better to start your week with goals that takes some time to adjust to be constructive. If you are at your best with running, you usually can't be told otherwise if people start to challenge your expertise because it will roll off you. Why should you let someone who has a different method of teaching make you feel that your time pushing ahead has not worked for you? For example, in a grocery store, there are so many things that make good customer service, that if you feel a question was misunderstood, you should not let it affect you negatively and mentally.

I can make choices for myself such as eating a healthy breakfast and turning off my computer at night that let me start my day and end my night well. When I trained at the gym, I would often spend four to five hours a day in the morning on a Sunday or one hour on Monday with various exercise classes and various long-distance treadmill runs to be seen as a normal person pushing themselves to their limits. Someone who tries to make a life for themselves can show others to do the same and start to make the choices that are needed for success.

In running as a means of exercise, a runner needs to see where they are in their fitness plan and make runs according to how they see they have the time to be fit. With having state of the art facility in gyms such as the 24 Hour Fitness, a runner is able to have an abundance of tools to exercise and either undertrain, train right, or overtrain their bodies. It is best to find a comfort zone that lets you have proper diet and exercise and time to enjoy your life. In seeing how races are organized, a runner needs to be able to take in the air they breathe normally.

With my experience of exercise at my local gym and by seeing the different styles in the members who exercise and the instructors who teach, it gave me my own edge and push that set myself apart because I put more time into my body for moral and self-esteem. Perhaps the push could exhaust myself, but a later time, I could see how the movements of runners that I haven't met made me a winner at the race because I talked about how I've trained and how I'm ready for the race.

Since you are in control of your body, you are the one who calls the shots. Every place of business is open for the customer to make a life for themselves, and if you go through the social pressure of questioning yourself or if other people question you about how much time is enough to train, you can see that people work together to find a suitable goal. People work together in all forms of running, and if a pack of runners near the start of a marathon finish together at the end, they are showing the running world that they accomplished their goal together.

In addition to spending four to five hours a day at the gym in the morning, I found other nights where I could do the same and found a way to taper my body to train well. My mom could drive to the gym in front of me to a yoga class at the local 24 Hour Fitness gym, and I'd notice in class how her feedback at the gym differed from home. At home, my mom could solve a puzzle, and I spend my time at home, work, and other places productively while letting my parents enjoy themselves.

In an enigma, an investor who wants to invest in stocks or bonds calls a money manager or stock broker to help them invest to make a long-term gain, but they don't earn money. In times of trading and the war Russia started with Ukraine, there are added enigmas that need to be solved, but while keeping your health alive with the resources you have, you can find your body keeping its shape.

After classes at the gym such as yoga, I would run on the treadmill for fifteen miles a night. During my running, I had headphones with music, and I interpreted stimuli through watching television, the gym team members, and the other members exercising. I felt mentally and physically better to the point that I enjoyed my time, and my GI doctor took note of how I was doing remarkably well, recovering from my dehydration from the 2017 LA Marathon.

There are training secrets that running can uncover such as how cyclists train to get through their miles as a runner runs. Oftentimes I've noticed that with indoor cycling, a person is going through rigorous training to cycle at a better pace and speed from other cyclists as they cycle their miles. A cyclist can cycle long tours or long rides as they train their body to work, and I've used this to run faster and healthier.

When a runner has a long distance to run, they often can see long roads ahead of them with many miles left to run. In the cycling world, a cyclist can see long distances or miles ahead of them, as my experience with indoor cycling at the gym showed me. Even with hundreds of miles run in a few days, there are cyclists that can shape reality within a few moments of indoor cycling or riding and catch a runner's progress in a different way. The challenge comes for the runner to be able to maintain glory in their miles run and a way catch the cyclist's glory and be able to ultimately maintain or run more miles with the same confidence.

Cycling can also help for marathon running because indoor cycling often gives a runner a sense of light when they train even though they are not running. It is similar to someone going to the mall and enjoying reading a book; when the person is causally doing something that they enjoy, they feel an urge to do more with themselves and shop. A runner is doing a different from of exercise than a cyclist who rides a bike. Cycling often lets a person ride a longer distance in one hour than running often does. The combination of cycling and running can give an athlete more sense of a physical comfort in many situations on a marathon course where they can now advance. After cycling, social interactions can make you adjust back to the mindset of a runner to enjoy both sports and make progress.

One hour of cycling in the gym on a Monday morning can come running twenty-one miles on a treadmill the night before to give me an edge of comfort to start off my week as other cyclists also have pleasant experiences to share in their rides. Mondays give you a new opportunity to start off your week, letting you feel your work was completed in your previous week and you can start fresh. It is similar in school when students gather together for classes; they are put in a class not often to who they want to be with but with people that have worked just as hard in similar roles to be able to learn together. When a person feels they are a stranger, they have found comfort with others; just as in marathons, most runners are there to race to the finish.

Oftentimes during a race expo, there are opportunities to take pictures of yourself by the vendors either with the race logo's backdrop or on three steps that are similar to when the runner finishes the race and earns first, second, or third place. The special thing about standing on steps or blocks that are given to either the first, second, or third place runners is that you can feel the endorphins running through your body just by stepping up on the steps and taking a selfie.

In the cycling world, they say that you can be welcome to the cycling world by either having experience through cycle classes, BMX biking, mountain biking, or any other form of cycling. Many cyclists become accustomed to it that they make it a habit to cycle whenever they can. At any point in time, a cyclist can change their goal to being a runner, and at any point, a runner can also add cycling into their schedule to improve their speed while running.

It can seem that with all the cyclists riding their bikes that all you need to do is step up some blocks in your running, and get first, second, or third place. For example, during a cycling class at a gym, you can look outside of the cycling class to see members of the gym stepping on a stair climber or lifting weights, as they exert energy to build their bodies and train at a higher level. In the Palos Verdes LaceUp Running Series, their photographers in the expo let you step up to the first, second, and third place steps for an Instagram picture, and after the race, the real winners were announced with their place and times, stepped up, were photographed, and rewarded the prize money and a plaque for their achievement. Running itself can often be the best form of training your body to run faster for a race to feel comfort and to not overload yourself.

The exercise classes at the gym let me see myself in the mirror from different angles, and I'd often have a marathon shirt on while the instructor gave me words of encouragement or told me to come on or that I can do it. In my mind, I was doing good enough, and I wanted to feel the success of running the previous night. By running a lot of miles each night, the next day made me believe more in myself and not to take the words of the instructors so seriously. Standards to qualify for an event for Olympic became a notion to understand, and people have seen me as a runner in some situations and in others they don't. It is similar to a person trying something new as they need to adapt to the stimuli to go with the flow.

It is a priority to get enough exercise in the day, work, and properly train to feel good relative to how others perceive me. My perception of maintaining a healthy lifestyle was to go to the gym although I'm not a member now and no longer attend the GX classes. Instead, I exercise with an assortment of workouts and maintain a healthy diet with the 24 Hour Fitness training app called Future at home, which is important for my sense of well-being in life.

As a runner in your journey, you will know when you feel that you have pushed your limits on your body or if you still have more effort to give. By staying within the rules of a race and being able to run hard and fast, you can find ways make it to the finish line when you felt it was hard. In the ultramarathon, the feedback that I got from some of the other runners definitely helped me to see it as an accomplishment.

"It was a beast" is what I heard from other runners, and my feelings of going to start the second marathon were also satisfactory as I knew I wasn't the only one taking on the challenge. The race itself is something that takes a lot of emotional willpower before and even after the race. When someone tells you something that you aren't prepared for, you can feel the same as you did as you felt beforehand by changing of your mental thinking to get to your goal.

The difference with being at the gym or work to running an ultramarathon can be large because in a sense, when you are running in an ultramarathon, you are going for a goal. While you are running the race, you can have a headlamp, a reflective vest, pepper spray or a whistle, a hat, a cell phone, and safety items whereas in a gym, you can see your locker with various items in it as you start to train.

It was after fifteen miles of running at the gym or twenty-one miles of running throughout the day that I considered it to be a success for myself in my struggle to progress as a person and an athlete. The journey in the gym can lead to many successes when a runner is able to gain an edge on how they see themselves. The reason that a lot of people have positive attitudes in life is that they are able to feel a comfort in themselves first. The instant when a runner finishes a run and later the exercises shows the world that they are an athlete as they gracefully have the power to settle into the society. After you race, if you are at a gym, you can feel your timing efforts from your marathon allow you to comfortably perform most exercises.

The way runners run in packs is also important to show as various volunteers work together to make a race. When volunteers or race directors set up their area before a race, they often have a lot of things to prepare for such as setting up aid stations for water or electrolytes, food or snacks, course markers, and emergency aid that are needed by the runners. The volunteers later clean up after the runners and themselves, and they leave the area they've worked after the race is finished. After the race, the neighborhood streets are reopened to the public, and there is a sense of rebuilding or peace. Oftentimes, the cars in streets use their horns as the runners try to cross the streets, and they are guided by the police officers.

Neighbors can read about the race in the newspaper the day after, and they are able to see what a positive thing the event was for the neighborhood. After the race, a runner can visit the area again and feel many impressions as they see traffic getting back to normal. One is a sense of calmness or an added ability to converse with people as they get back to their lives. A runner can use the news to improve their running by reading the event and the successful runners. Another is that a runner can remember more if they see their family at the finish line after a race because the race is fresh in their heads, and by taking pictures, they have a clear image of their loved ones.

Running can be improved from your fastest level, as I was told that I need to learn how to run by a trainer at a gym. The visual aspects a runner gets or cues throughout their journey are immense, and the way to get a better idea of the running is through using the constructive criticism or advice from others to your advantage. When a runner gets a medal, they can feel successful, but people who are heavy into fitness or even random gym members might not know your accomplishments. There is a moment where you see a customer entering a place where you can sense an appreciation in most instances. When you are in a similar situation in a distant time away, you can often sense a circle in the appreciation that can turn toward your ego, but keep your ego under control. The journey of the runner is to strive for their bodies to feel conditioned and able to adapt to many situations in an affirmative manner.

Runners can improve their awareness with mental activities, such as reading, that are light and easy. If a runner continually challenges himself to feel positive thoughts and stimuli in the outside world, then the runner can grow as a person. When the runner is going through various parts of a city, he can be able to find a technique of thinking and enthusiasm that helps him be happier.

In the course of a marathon, try to find a technique to practice ways to acknowledge feedback from others. Near the end of a marathon, a runner can get through the race with a feeling that they have a lot more to give and that they have the energy to run faster. With anything from hearing a volunteer say, "Good job," "You're almost there," and "Champion," if you tell them thanks or at least feel with your heart that it was a positive experience, you'll feel better mentally and physically.

At the end of a race, the runner can tell themselves that they have more energy, but they have given so much in the race that they can just decide it was enough. This is how I often feel near the end of the race with minor aches or sore legs. I can sense the environment at the finish line, and if I sense it near the twenty-first mile, then I can tell myself to run my fastest before I finish. When I feel my body has surpassed my normal comfort level, there is something inside of me telling me I am confidently almost done with the race and to keep running. Another is that feeling of glory because I know I am going to comfortably finish and get a medal and enjoy some time to relax and have fun. If I were to listen to my body and walk or spend time stretching, I could lose time, but I feel fit enough to finish my race.

A new ground can be broken through visualizing the finish line before you are there. In my experience with running and working to improve my pace, my body feels like it can get past the point where I felt tired or exhausted. For example, by the time the twenty-fourth mile comes, it can be reassuring to know you'll finish with an adequate pace and get the needed sleep afterward. The psychological benefits of feeling an elated, euphoric state or a runner high can be a form of therapy for people with addiction or depression.

After a marathon ends, you can go back into society feeling like a holiday came or a day off work as you prepared enough to race well and not relive it since the race is over and the work was well worth it. For example, when a runner orders an item online such as picture or online photo of himself or herself crossing the finish line, they can see messages from the merchant such as, "Wow, great work out there," which gives a feeling of relief that the race is done.

The real-world experience of relaxing with family and friends after a marathon can make more focused at work with employees in your company who also accomplish goals and advance in their careers. You can find a middle ground to relax and get a peace of mind from your accomplishment. When a person climbs the corporate ladder to become a CEO, they have to put a lot of work and time to get that goal.

My breathing can increase its rhythm while I breath hard through my mouth comfortably. Later I will try to catch myself to breathe through my nose and breathe out through my mouth every few seconds. People live at their comfort level in their everyday life supporting the runners, and the expectations of others when they try to push you harder or tell you that you're not pushing enough can naturally be overcome by running a little harder and talking to other volunteers on the course.

The social interactions a runner can experience in the community can come from a variety of places such as from friends, neighbors, or people who work for the community. There are many instances after runs when the legs get soar or tired and you need to use cream or ointment at night to prevent cracking. When the night winds down, you can prepare for the next day by working, showering, or eating a healthy meal. The runner can plan goals for the different days of the week and the time of day to improve productivity and satisfaction. I am able to experience a wind in my strides as I run that makes me feel that I'm giving my body's maximum effort when running. My body's ability to rest after a race or go to work or at home shows me that I'm resting in a place that is different from the course where I ran.

In marathons, there's usually a straight course or a windy path with hills that leads you to the finish line. With the course, the race organizers make a way to challenge the runner with various steeper hills and trails that can be exhausting. After getting through markers or miles, the runner can see volunteers or authorities guiding others to show and push you to run faster, and it has led you to the right place.

In the world of buying and selling items for yourself or to make a profit, one can visit a convenience store, pharmacy, or any other place to help you to a point to where you are both satisfied. A runner can also mentally push through a run, which gives them an advantage when they are finished and shop in a store and use their knowledge confidently to get items that they usually need. The real edge is being able to see yourself and put your goals in place as a runner to earn a real sense of earned confidence when it comes to the everyday tasks that you do. After a virtual run, a runner gets a grace period after their work or run to the time they input their results in when they get their medal.

The unique aspect of many races is that there are alternate ways to post your time, and some races allow you to post your virtual run before getting your medal and swag. Some races allow you to run your race well before the race date and hold on to your time before submitting your results when the window is open. Some races require you to run your virtual race around a certain time frame because they accept race results in a certain time frame. The experience of getting your medal varies from race to race often because of the time frame to submit your results.

A runner can train better by being consistent to find the things that make them happier and build that from their discovery. Training every day lets you learn new ways to remember things that you forgot, and you can pick up the pieces. Once you define the pieces that you need help with, you can start to feel the sense of growth and go to the root of the issue.

The normal human body form with naturally defined abs, a built physique, and a healthy mind can always serve as a role model to where you are today. As I was going through grade school to intermediate school to high school, I found that the body and mind needed to match each other in the culture I lived in. In my culture, there is a lot of family togetherness, which helps a person to grow up with a variety of people and integrate well for a better chance of success.

Freedom in America looks to the right of people to control their lifestyle without interference from the government or organized authority. If you've worked hard to find happiness or the American Dream to find yourself on a route in life where you eat food that make you overweight or rick disease, try to build a body in accordance to other standards such as an athlete or fitness role model.

I first started weight lifting in 1995, and my urge was to follow a type of diet and exercise where I would eat El Pollo Loco for a meal and try to count calories for the first time. I experimented with MET-Rx meal replacement bars and protein shakes and order large quantities and eat suitably. There is a social stigma that can get the body out of its comfort zone by watching the types of food to eat if they are unnatural, which can make the body change its shape quickly, which is what happened to my body.

My body became a lot larger in the chest and bicep area, but I still was able to maintain healthy goals and a liking to material possessions such as watches. In the gym, no matter where you are in your workout or how you choose your food, others are there putting in more time than you and eating differently. Some make you feel like you are in the right place, but that there is more you need to do to get to your goals. By running miles on a treadmill with the guide of a trainer, then you can learn the basics such as the speed to train at or you're incline to make you burn calories. It felt similar to the process of learning a new trick or sport, and I became comfortable with putting the treadmill on a certain speed and knowing when to turn it off and how to grip the heart rate sensors using my watch.

People can live their lives according to the career paths they chose, and some haven't used treadmill training. A professional can learn how to handle a lot of situations in the work force and be a runner, and his goals can be achieved with running. The body's form goes through many stages when running as it can get leaner and stronger with the more miles, and the mind also follows by accepting stimuli well. The more experience someone has in a gym setting with the various workout equipment, the more their paths chosen become understood.

A goal of better interactions with others about an issue where you have to run and be considered can be put into a different type of perspective through public speaking such as Toastmasters International. The body and mind can come together to have the person see things inside themselves that they haven't seen and be put in another positive perspective. For example, when a person grows up and hears about the things that various presidents have achieved, they can feel that they have a life that needs to be lived or that the things they are doing are in line with how strong they believe they are.

There are a lot of factors that make the runners successful, and each factor works with one another to make the person feel as though they are in a better position than they were a few minutes ago. When a runner is able to talk through feedback from another person, he or she is able to take a course of action. For example, the option to buy food before or after a marathon can be healthy or unhealthy, but since you have the mindset of performing well in the race, the people you talk to will encourage you to eat healthy.

The various days and nights that a runner puts in to his practice should set him up for success. The real-life aspect of communicating with people and relating to others can go in a circle if you don't keep reasonable intentions. A runner improves his training usually on his own time with effort to change from within and understand how his body can perform superiorly and run quicker.

A runner can be a better person in society by having a tough attitude, and oftentimes their donations can go toward special causes. A tough attitude makes a person strong because it's needed to push yourself further during a marathon. The runner gets smarter and his desire comes from many places but ultimately from within.

When a person goes shopping or to exercise, there are always places that people can store their bicycles. Even in a university or grocery stores, people can lock their bikes outside so they can go about their business or shop or walk.

As a runner, you can often experience various challenges or surprises when you talk at the expo to outside vendors, merchants, or people at their business who work within the community. I found the edge I have when running builds my character to live comfortably among various athletes such as cyclists, walkers, and hikers. The psychological edge that a runner can get through an ultramarathon or a long running event is very sensational, and often it becomes easier to maintain a balanced lifestyle with a stable career. In the real world, you can further your education and learning more in school, and my choice to educate myself with a master of business administration degree has shown me how to get ahead in the world with various people who are at different places in their work and social life.

The more a person learns while they run, they become smarter; and with running more, you can add a level of athletics in your lifestyle. It is similar to a person who wants to pursue a PhD in their field of studies. With more education, the individual could perhaps be at a different level of income or be in a new field. There are various research jobs that a person, such as myself, can get to have $20,000 a year with a PhD, and many other opportunities can arise to reach another plateau.

Changes in perceptions of how people in the food service, culinary, gas, or any other business view the runner can be for the better. In my experience with talking to various merchants, vendors, gas stations, and places of business, it seems as though by placing your successes and achievements aside and being yourself, you can often feel appreciated and respected by them. Other times, it seems as though you still have to look out for yourself and your own happiness to be heard. In running, you have time to reflect on how situations have treated you and find ways to develop smarter through your connections.

Deep breaths at the start of the race can help you feel more natural and condition your body to avoid pushing itself too hard. Runners can see the sun while running because their body is moving to the weather. While a person is at work, before the sun sets, there is a method of unwinding and not getting sidetracked to take care of your body to prepare yourself for your next run. When running in the sun, you can visualize the sun over your head and apply sunscreen when needed to sooth your skin.

A new goal can be understanding a different perception of someone else's plan for it to help you. It can change your behavior to make yourself more accepting to certain diets and training plans. COVID-19 has made changes to how some people live, and social distancing while running and wearing a face mask at the start of the race is mandatory, often if you aren't vaccinated. With the current events in the world today, some people question whether some of the news is a hoax or if it is really worth abiding by.

I have the time to run marathons virtually and physically, and I kept a positive vision and change in light of the news. One way of seeing the world I always knew is by looking at the cautions I've placed in areas. I say to myself just in case I do not have the time to exercise, I still want to feel healthy. What would it be like if there was no work to do? Some of these events have taken place today where I now have the time to sleep to the time that works for me. My various jobs such as a delivery driver with Uber Eats or a courtesy clerk with Ralphs make my present time seem special to look forward to travel to marathons.

In the real world of working a nine-to-five job or spending your time at an office building in a cubicle where you do not have the time to do other things is something that many do when they don't want to. Throughout my life with work, I felt that a lot of the hours I put in should give me more income than I got. Now I feel gratitude for the present while some things could go back to normal. It is similar to the hours I spent at the gym running and in GX classes where a person works and perceives your experience, and later you feel like you can relax with a family member that perceives things differently.

The way that I exercise in a gym has made me realize that there are many mirrors, and by having a mirror in front of me while running, I can watch my form and make adjustments as needed.

The Persian culture differs from others, and my parents view my lifestyle as someone who grew up in Iran, and I grew up in America. Most cultures are able to adapt to others, and in the United States, people are accepting of most cultures. There have been culture clashes that made it much harder for many minorities to coexist. My parents are high achievers because they were successful in their fields before they retired. My vision in the morning is one of success to be able to work, live at home, recover, and run. My parents have had a lot of success, and my eyes adjust later in the day after communicating with them because they love me. My parents live their own lives and lifestyles as they let me love in my own ways.

Running has a goal that is accomplished by finishing, and it gives me time to adjust to find new goals and find life to be fun. Recently, my aunt traveled with me to Iran, and I wanted to run outside my relative's home, and I wasn't supposed to show off my American running clothes because it could make a scene in the neighborhood while I ran.

A person often lives life according to standards learned from their parents or in schools. First, a person attends school. Later he or she gets a job, and later the person can decide to go back to school to learn more, work other jobs, or even buy a home. When a runner pays a registration fee for a race, they are paying to be able to participate, and rarely are runners paid to run unless they are sponsored or have advertising deals with companies. When a person finishes school and gets a college degree, they are then put into the real world of working, and life can change for the better with job opportunities.

When a runner pays a fee to join a race, they later find a way to travel to the race or they can just race virtually from start to finish. In the situation where you have parents that you can look up to at home, it can be a start of a journey to run faster by pinpointing the areas that you can work on. I found it useful not to compare yourself with others but to have your own path that you are successful.

When a child looks into their parents' eyes, they feel a sense of trust and belonging. At every age, a child can look into their parents' eyes and feel that they have more and more to accomplish. Or they can get to a point where they do not have to do everything to try to live under their parents' rules or not to do something that they do not want to just to please their parents. The story of a child growing up to be a runner is something that the child goes through with various barriers to see the other side of life, which is filled with joy and appreciation.

A disease can alter your own way of life so that you are no longer capable to performing the way you had been and must be avoided. My situation has also been altered by doctors because my mental health has been something that my psychiatrist and other doctors have assisted me with. Chronic paranoid schizophrenia has been changed to in chronic paranoid schizophrenia in partial remission. By being able to get out of the 1 percent of the population with the disease, it is something that I'm proud of and attribute a lot of it to my running.

When you see examples of people who are successful in life, it can be helpful to have a role model. With certain role models, you are able to set a goal or use them as your mentor to show you how to achieve what you want. In the American Dream, every citizen of the United States should have an equal chance to attain success and wealth through hard work, determination, and initiative. A person often works hard in their careers to have a house, a well-paying career in a field that is admirable, and often a husband or wife to abide by. With running, the dream can be built in a similar way, as the runner has shown that he or she knows a course well enough to be able to complete the run and enjoy the benefits they get from it. The feelings of joy and gratitude can last for a few weeks up to the next race or stay with you because by completing a marathon, you have been able to accomplish something that 99 percent of the population can't.

Uncle Sam is a common national image of the US Federal government that came in 1812 named for Samuel Wilson. America uses

Uncle Sam for many reasons, and as tax purposes a novel idea for people to follow is "I want you to pay your taxes" or "I want you for the US Army." In the running world, Uncle Sam has meaning to me because I expect something positive from my interactions with people. Uncle Sam is someone who wants Americans to work hard and live the American Dream of having a reputable career and a higher level of income.

Many races have routes through affluent places that people live, as runners race through and overcome pressure. A runner can run through many courses and feel that they have a strong character as a runner because they've faced the social pressures that many successful people have. People have a common way of greeting one another and communicating in the real world, and oftentimes, someone tries to help out another person through listening and helping.

A runner high can be a feeling of happiness often at the finish line of a run you want to have for a pleasant memory. Just as an investor buys gold to hold onto it for as long as possible to make a profit or a stock holder that buys a security and holds it long enough to earn a profit, the happiness gained from an event can stay with you for a long time. There are ways to further enjoy the benefits of the runs at home or other places such as by looking at a picture of yourself in the run or you're having your own finisher's certificate or medal.

A runner should not snap at others in the places he or she visits because your emotions may be intense, and if you keep a happy attitude, you'll escape the urge to give negative feedback. In life, there are many people who often feed off others to make themselves feel better, and when you identify that situation, you'll navigate through it with ease.

Sales people on the telephone often try to give you an offer that is not in your best interests; many of these are scams to avoid. The sales people could often drain the energy out of you and take for themselves as they try to sell you a product, but you can just not accept those calls or block the caller as a solution. When a runner carefully plans for a race and he or she later completes the race, it's a reason to feel good. There are many ways to lose touch with the work you did that got you there because of the natural feeling to just let yourself enjoy the moment.

In life, when there is money around such as in a restaurant or store, there are salespeople who have busy lifestyles and need to communicate to satisfy the customer. When I buy something, often I search to find meaning in a situation after it was sold because with peace of mind of buying something, you know you didn't waste your money. I will usually get a receipt for a purchase when I feel like it is necessary and try to end the conversation on a pleasant note. Just as when a runner keeps their persistence with making to the next mile, they are given praise by volunteers for doing a good job.

A runner's time is valuable when they feel their effort was given. After the race, the clock was finished for the runner, and they can hear the announcer say his or her name and where they are from and even hear a word of encouragement. Once the runner crosses the finish line, they have completed the event and the event is over, but they can add satisfaction by knowing they can view their results online later and order items that are needed.

Most of the time, the course is closed after a race until the next race. The course usually has nearby areas closed for the race itself for the runners to run their route. The interactions that the runner has while running the race and the feelings that can arise are there as a learning experience for what the person experiences in their daily life. Once the runner gets back into their lives, they find that have picked up at a place that feels comfortable for them. Perhaps the runner can now find a way to handle social pressure that they've felt before in a more positive way. Today, there are stereotypes and prejudices that people see but do not act on it, and after finishing a race, the runner can naturally make a positive social movement.

A person has twenty-four hours in a day where they have time to sleep, rest, and live their day, and if you add running to it, your day goes better because you have added more activity. There often gifted people in certain areas of life that allow them to be happier, make more money, and be more charismatic. If someone has these traits, they can find it easier to accomplish certain tasks in life and ways to achieve the success.

I have found that it is easier to deal with people at a customer service level because I have the ability to comprehend other people's situations with ease in a way that makes me feel more comfortable with them. It is a feeling of well-being, but it often does not stop there because one customer after the next can lessen your energy as you need to be aware of scams. After communicating to another person, you can see that they, too, have aspirations. When running on a course, you can see that you could be giving all of your energy to run the event to finish. In the customer service level, it is said that the customer comes first and what they say is right, but when you're running, it's just you and the road to the finish line.

When dealing with the customer, you need to listen to their needs and help them the best you can to not lose them. The way running involves your needs is that you need to be able to have a sense of how hard your body can push in an event for you to not injure or dehydrate yourself. Once you know your body and its limits, you can set a better pace for yourself and be able to know when you are pushing too much or not enough. Injuries can occur with running because of its high-impact nature, and with changes in your running volume or pace, you can develop more. You can find that your muscles can cramp and you can take steps to minimize injuries by warming up before exercises, eating a well-balanced diet, and allowing yourself time to recover.

In the running world when there is a race, you see time is on your side as the clock starts and you participate with groups of runners that often run in packs in order from start to finish. The way an atmosphere such as the gym helps a runner is that the runner can see that time is on their side with the various exercises that they perform in addition to the weights lifted, treadmill running, and classes participated in, but they are not being timed like in a marathon. This shows that although it could be possible to exercise for twenty-four hours straight or even more, your body would eventually feel the burden of having malnutrition and being exhausted. Although it is possible to work for twenty-four hours, it is probably not in your best interest because you would feel tired and not be able to take care of your body the right way. A runner can feel more appreciated for the reactions that they see in other because if you see yourself having a fun time, you can see the fun in others without overdoing yourself and giving yourself time to relax.

The running world often can make a runner feel surprised in the outside world because once you're done running and going back to your normal life, you can find yourself needing to adjust to social situations differently. When interactions occur that can seem confusing, a runner can turn back the clock and answer questions. In my experience with running, I've found a way to solve problems that is easy if done right. Since each marathon gives a description of the start point, start time, expo time, and dates along with course information, it gives me a sense of knowing what to expect.

If this is carefully planned, a runner can use these directions to help them get ahead and be more prepared when they experience questions. There is a lot to learn with running while you are not running. For example, when I am at a restaurant or place to eat that has a menu, I feel comfortable when I order food because I have time to look at the menu. I've noticed that a lot of merchants do not give me the luxury of looking at the menu when I am picking up food for Uber Eats as a delivery driver because we are more focused on me picking up the food and safely delivering it to the customer. These are enigmas in time because of persistence and my desire to become a better runner and all-around person.

Just as a runner enters a field of hundreds of runners in a marathon, a place of business with vendors can make you feel that you have to learn how to do more than run. In athletics, there are many sports that a person can master such as basketball, baseball, or football. If a runner enters a group of cyclists, he or she can learn how they tend to cycle and also pack together to have a sense of comradery to adapt to the outside world. There are many ways to gear up riding a bike and many ways to enjoy a smooth ride.

If you master your own sense of how much your body can endure, then you can also master the feeling when another person makes you feel a little bit untrained. In the professional world of business, there are countless people who try to make you feel a sense that you need more. I have experienced this with spending money.

For example, if I feel a little bit uncomfortable at an OC fair after an OC Fair 5K, I would play more games because I know that is the way that I can earn a prize. Although a little bit awkward, it is the same as someone ordering more and more pizza because they feel like they are making a relationship with the cook or chef. However, in reality, you are making yourself a little bit looser and flabbier in the stomach area because you've realized that you've gained a few pounds.

The experience a runner has after feeling everything is well and accomplished can change instantly by other people's perceptions or where they are in a day. An example is the age-grade results that are given to marathon runners. Every race has an age-grade percentage of how the runner did relative to other runners. If a race is a Boston Marathon qualifier, there is also a BQ percent given to the runner to see how close they are to qualifying to run in Boston.

When I enter a store working for Uber Eats or a place where there is a younger worker, who is perhaps at a different socioeconomic level in school, work ethic, and location, they can perceive my interactions as awkward, but they are doing their jobs, giving me the food I need to deliver. When there is music in a shopping center, it creates a reality that lets customers feel well with their experience in shopping, and when a person wants to try new things, such as a new job or a new sport, they adjust their schedule. The part of the change that you should focus on is giving yourself perspective of how you've improved and where you are with your running. Some people might be a little slower with their routines while others might not produce as much, and with a change in your routine, you can make adjustments to your running lifestyle.

A person in high school has the social pressure of going to the prom or trying to figure out what path they want to take in life to feel normal. People need to make decisions, and oftentimes the outcome might not be good for some people. In the world today, most people believe in God as a source of trust to communicate and function well in the day. This standard is something that the world holds well, but if you live your life with a purpose that lets you try a little bit harder, you can find running goals to achieve.

Perhaps you feel like you don't have the social intelligence to handle an experience or task that is given, but there are ways to make the effort come to your favor with extra effort on your behalf. In running an event, the feeling of gratitude comes usually before, during, and after the event, which is healthy. At this point, the person can start to plan for their next race, and the training can start sooner or later, depending on how long your body needs to recover.

The way to question and second-guess some things in life is a natural occurrence, but by going through life events with confidence and a goal in mind, you are going to do much better. In running, consistently having a plan toward keeping yourself with composure and confidence is also needed for you to implement well. A runner should be able to see themselves as capable of acting well at all times. For example, when I drive to various restaurants to pick up items for customers' orders, I can see many cyclists that are riding a long distance with cycling gear for their sport.

When a person drives a car, their body is in a place that is more stationary than a cyclist who pedals fast. When a cyclist is near me or a runner is jogging while I am driving on a hill, I see how the weather plays in role in keeping me active and alert and how most people find ways to exercise. If it is 2:00 p.m. in the day and I feel that I have a race coming up the next day and I need to train, I can do so with better confidence because of my workday. I can later go for a run in the evening or late at night and see the whole road ahead of me and also see the that I have confidence in keeping myself able to run a long distance.

When a marathon comes that a runner has planned for and a runner is in the twentieth mile of the race, the runner can get a sense of encouragement and motivation to run at a faster pace. The runner can pick up some social cues they see from volunteers and the person at the race doing their jobs. The human body and mind are always interpreting things from the outside world to stay encouraged. There are many road signs in route to various places in a race and many ways that a runner can relax after the race, such as by going to a restaurant, going to a store, or even exercising.

The runner can build themselves to be brave in times that they perhaps weren't before. The same comes in my experience running in marathons where throughout the race, I tend to see familiar places on a course because I have experience in the run and I know the route and places to go. For example, the San Francisco Marathon has altered their course recently, but I have a sense of where the landmarks and where to run. Naturally my mind creates endorphins, and I'm able to run with a runner high or a sense of euphoria that is natural because my brain is producing endorphins. The feelings of well-being come, and I'm able to see other runners near me running just as well, or even better than me, and I can sense how some of my doubts or struggles with the outside world can change for the better.

With the early miles on the races such as the thirteenth or sixteenth mile of a marathon, there is a time period when a runner can already see some of the faster runners have finished their race and they are now at part of the course with their medal to watch or help others finish. My experience with seeing runners on their way to the finish line is that I usually have seven to ten miles left. These front runners get cheers, and I can see the work and fitness level that was put forth, and it motivates me to see myself as a winner. The faces of the runners show me signs of encouragement because I can tell that they are almost finished with the race and they often have looks of experience and of winners. Oftentimes, I know with all the training I've done that I can relate with their stamina and running effort.

When people with different intentions look to my confidence and motivation when I visit restaurants or store, things said can seem confusing or out of place, but with my work effort, I'll get my job done. For example, when I visit a restaurant for the first time, I can see a menu, and I have the choice to order food for myself in addition to pick up someone else's order. In a race, I have the choice to push myself a little bit harder to feel less energy at later parts in the race. Runners should conserve their energy up until twenty-two miles to run at a pace where they can finish.

Time management in marathons, business, and homes comes in many forms. For example, a plan to get enough sleep can help a runner go to bed at a certain time for a certain number of hours of sleep for the best performance. Most runners have a sense of time management because they've made it to the race and are prepared to run with others.

Time is on your side if you plan your day, week, month, or year better than the previous one. If issues arise with a health-care provider, I can plan for myself to still be seen for my appointments by researching options. It is important to get a certain amount of rest every day to drive safe and communicate well at work and at home. It is important to be in good terms with your overall health every day and every time you talk through therapy and appointments. Through proper time management, I can look out for myself get ahead mentally and financially to try to make my career work and advance.

With an equal amount of time given to my employers, I'm able to earn have a surplus of income at the end of the month. For example, if I start working for Uber Eats with a delivery at 10:00 a.m. and later I have work at the grocery store Ralphs from 2:30 p.m. to 10:30 p.m., that leaves me with an adequate source of income. I could end up getting home at midnight if I'd make more time for the Uber Eats delivery at 10:30 p.m., but I wouldn't sleep too much. With proper planning, eating a healthy meal, and taking care of myself by exercising or running at the start of the day, I can sleep six to eleven hours a night. I could work for Uber Eats at any time of the day since the work delivering the food is around the clock, but it's better to get the rest that's needed for the next day.

This scenario of working around the clock lets me communicate some things to my psychologist and psychiatrist differently because any changes that I want to make could be discussed. I'm able to talk to my parents about anything, and I look to help them in the day. In one aspect, I feel the sense of comfort because I can listen to my parents and converse with them just as well as doctors or therapists. The day often changes because of the different social interactions and conversations with my parents.

A runner can sense many things on a course that discourage them such as an injury due to lack of training. For example, the government is a man-made entity that exits for citizens to live with, and we must follow the law and standards the government gives us.

People often need legal help to relax after they get a settlement or compensation. In a marathon, I feel comfort to see the time of the day and weather change and that the right choices were made to choose the race.

Some marathons start at 5:30 a.m. or 6:00 a.m., which makes my mind sharp for me to leave my house by 3:00 a.m., depending on how far the race is, to catch a shuttle. When the sun is still not out, you could feel tired to be the only one awake at your house before leaving, but it can be a wonderful change to be willing and fully awake with the community to experience the day ahead. The drive to the race can often feel tiring as time seems slow because of boredom, tension, and difficulty concentrating on many things to get to start the race. The tension could be eased through therapy, exercising, work in my daily life, and with adequate rest.

The car drive to a marathon is often interesting for me because my focus is to not get drowsy on my way to the race and back home. While driving to the event, I can feel a lot of reactions of other drivers as I try to keep my attention on one thing, such as road, music playing, and my signaling. I prepare well enough for the event by having a map on where to go and by being on time for the event. When the day after the race comes, the feeling of time while driving home also changes from the run to a certain feeling of joy from yourself and others for completing an event. I can focus on driving safe and have a positive attitude and full amount of energy for the race, which are essential to plan heading into the run. People stay informed and get by often by reading the newspaper and watching television, which differs from actually being in public with people because you can exercise your mind as you interact with people.

When getting to the parking lot, there are always fellow runners that have parked around the same time as you and that are also getting prepared with other people to get to the race, which can make you feel that you are not alone. There is a feeling of comfort in a way because you can give yourself a sense of satisfaction by seeing other people who are going to get involved in a fun sport. The more people that you see around you and the more you are able to give your body the final pushes before the race, the better off you are in your journey to have a fine race.

The mind can change with improved interaction while staying active to let you live with more self-reliance toward family. My parents and I exist well, but they are the homeowners of the house, and we can have mixed reactions after a full night's sleep or after a healthy meal to find a balance. I make eye contact and converse with my parents to feel justified with my choices, and they are proud of me.

I understand that the American culture differs from the Persian one in many terms such as in marriage ideals. In the Persian culture, there are numerous standards and expectations that a family gives a child to adhere to before adulthood such as going to school, owning a home, having a job, and being married, and many in Iran and America can continue to live with family and relatives as long as they can. In the culture of Iran, the family is very close to each other and many live and play together from childhood to adulthood. Oftentimes the expectations are easier to accomplish, and oftentimes they can be harder. Improved sleep has helped me to see the time living and talking to my parents as time is well spent.

A Persian family living in America can be just as successful as some of the wealthier families, and a Shah princess recently purchased one of the two most expensive houses in Beverly Hills to show how Americans and Iranians can live similar lifestyles.

Through adjusting to the real-world ways that people live and work, a person can integrate into the society and learn various values that have been taught to them. In my situation after graduating with my MBA from CSUDH, it was one of the hardest and most rewarding experiences, adjusting to the lifestyle from studying in school to working in the real world. By attending various events and participating in local clubs and through the support with therapy, speaking groups such as Toastmasters International, and different jobs, it made the transition easier. My parents did not pressure me to uphold a standard of getting good grades for my master of business administration degree from California State University Dominguez Hills. I decided to use my time to study well in school and get good grades, and I earned a 3.81 GPA to feel that I comfortably passed my classes.

The training that a runner can do at their home such as fifteen-minute workouts at the start of the day or core exercises with the abdomen can help you perform better in a race. My mom recently told me that I didn't train enough for my recent 2020 Los Angeles Marathon, and it made me feel a little bit startled. I was anticipating a positive response after my run, and it was, but my time was not under five hours. I finished the marathon, and I felt that I did train enough and I was satisfied, which is important. A runner can see themselves winning a marathon if they are satisfied with their level of activity, time, and training.

A runner can make the change to have a positive self-image of themselves by finding out that you must love yourself before you can love others. In the running world, there can be competition in being on time and social pressures to sort out the things that make you feel uncomfortable. For example, if a certain diet didn't work for me and I gained fat instead of muscle, the diet must be changed to help me move forward.

There can be many obstacles that a person must overcome to become successful, and you might have additional boundaries that your parents didn't have. For example, in the quest to make a lot of money, there are some paths such as an MBA, CPA, medical degree, or law degree that have works for most and other paths such as owning your own business that give a person more potential to earn money. As in a career, a runner can put out their best foot forward to meet people before the race to run and recover properly. After a long run that goes many places, the body replenishes with rest to recover its lost energy levels.

An athlete is a person who is proficient in sports and exercise and has a way of keeping a high level of energy and needs rest. For example, when an athlete drives to school or work or travels, the road can take a toll on the body and rest stops are needed. The scenery on the roads can be beautiful, and at your stop, you can see people cross the streets.

As an athlete, you're trained in running, which requires an amount of strength and stamina to participate in with various feedback given from volunteers before and after the race. With effort-based running, you let your perceived effort be your guide instead of worrying about the time it takes to do a segment of the run.

Now with the effort given and seeing a volunteer give you water, it serves as a motivation for you to cross the finish line. A volunteer will hand you a medal or ask you what kind of food you want such as flavor of a granola bar or a banana to help you recover. The shift from running a marathon to a recovery run or a short run at an easy pace can help you continue to train safely.

When a person finds satisfying work that pays them well, they should take the new lifestyle and put their effort in the new job. In the real world, some barriers that are often difficult to surpass are home ownership, a prestigious career, a beautiful house, or earning an advanced degree. These barriers are often overcome by persistence in an effort to get to a higher level in life. For example, a person can spend countless hours preparing to pass an exam and they pass or countless hours in a job to earn their pay rent and they pay.

A runner can train with three types of runs—speed work, long slow distance, and recovery runs—to be able to see the next mile and avoid a cramp in the stomach or foot. These long slow distance runs promote your form and can be at a constant pace of a low intensity over a lengthy duration meant to minimize fatigue and risk of injury.

In a demanding profession such as doctor or lawyer, it requires a lot of physical and mental effort with the public, and you are often faced with long hours and need to plan your diet to avoid hunger and make moral decisions. A runner can set goal of their own pace and the advanced runner can plan for a twenty-mile run and conserve their energy until they have reached their goal.

A runner can find a rhythm in their lives through listening to the public or by reading the guide that welcomes you to the race by the city. You can see a light in the end of the tunnel as you get to the finish line. When the volunteers cheer you on, they are supporting your efforts and the cities as they guide you to be happier and fruitful in your run to the finish line. A well-balanced runner can absorb the stimuli and handle the obstacles that can come in a course. Proper preparation can be wearing the right clothing before the race, having a charger for my cell phone in case the battery dies, having ibuprofen in case I need it, and having a footpad in case my foot hurts. Runners often get exhausted and fatigued and need to drop out of the race because of being overheated or dehydrated, which mostly can be avoided through slower running to build your foundation to run faster and longer.

Deep breathing, positive self-talk, staying hydrated, and doing your own thing are rules to remember when running because whether you're running or racing, if you run at your own pace, you'll run healthier and make safer decisions. When the mind has a challenge, a person can use common sense to know their place in a run and a runner who is usually one of hundreds in a race you know you've paid for, and you can love your run.

More peace of mind is to keep it down while running or don't be so loud as you discuss with others about what contributed your success. If you have a friend that you know and you make it to the finish line with them, you can find yourself in a guarded area with many spectators standing and looking for their loved ones.

In these moments, the runner can watch their steps with their body, mind, and thoughts to find ways to take in glory. A runner can also feel accomplished if they aim fluids carefully as they drink because many times, drinks spill on the floor, on your bib, or on your clothes and needs to be dried or cleaned up. After a race and when it's time leave and go and you've noticed that you have a stink in your clothes from your race, you can comfortably go back to the moment where it started and learn of a way to prevent it. Friends often understand and confide in you for the hours of training and effort put in for your race, and if you dress well, you'll feel a sense of fulfillment.

In the running world, you can share stories about your activities that make you feel ready without comparing yourself and being in competition. The way to go in a race is to have mental focus on your goals in the run so you have a clearer path and aren't sidetracked by the various spectators on the streets. If you feel in place and accept others the way they are and forgive the people who hurt you without dwelling into the past, you can gain composure and focus on the course ahead of you.

The journey of running helps you find success, health, and satisfaction by meeting others with similarities; just as in any conversation, the two parties want to find something in common to discuss. Runners can constantly work on themselves to experience positive or negative reactions. The more positivity in the reaction, the more the runner begins to appreciate themselves and run better. A runner can avoid redlining from knowing that they are running at a maximum effort to not breakdown before the race finishes. Meeting experienced runners who have run many races at a gym, grocery store, while driving, or at a public place such as a restaurant can let you look forward to more success in your runs.

A speedster is a runner that runs in a group often with friends and is fast, and as an endurance monster, I'm someone who has run a lot of races close together including long runs and my objective to train at a better level from before the race. I've often run a race in a series and comfortably made it back home and sealed the feeling with ordering a finisher picture from the race. Often people wear their singlets at the gym or other places with pride that they've completed the race and are in public now and feel some attention given to them by team members at a gym. I'm also a combo runner because I perform well in all my workouts fairly well, either short or fast or long or slow. When I wear my singlet at the gym or at a public place after the race, it is fun to wear it proudly again in another workout or run.

When a person wants to run for president of the United States, they must be a natural born citizen, be the age of thirty-five, and have lived in the United States for fourteen years to go through a tremendous amount of work to be elected. The most athletic president was Gerald Ford, who was also a runner. President Obama played basketball well, and Herbert Hoover had a sport named after him, hoover-ball.

There are many societies that often form a culture and form ideas and social behaviors to make one society distinct from another. Running can let you handle the social pressures of how society operates. In a running club or running, you are part of a wide-ranging institution focusing on running and oriented toward the sport and leisure of running and track and field. Being athletic is part of the most successful people's lives.

In my experience with reading and getting better rest, I've found an interest in some areas of politics such as how the president of the United States handles situations and how I can also keep an optimistic perspective as a person who was not born in this country to live life equally with others.

In the journey of getting to the starting line of a run, there are often ways that runners can reserve their parking spaces with paying a fee and later being able to park at a certain time in the lot. The earlier a runner gets to the lot, the more chance he or she has on being able to start on time and communicate socially about race ahead.

Consumers in society expect business to constantly provide exceptional experience, similar to a runner using their skills to expect an entertaining marathon. Since of young age I've been at school, I entered restaurants and other public places to form an idea of a profession to pursue, and today I make choices that give me a competitive edge in the world. A paradox a runner can feel is the change of their efforts given to training for an event to how they actually perform in the event.

A boxer can build so much experience in himself to feel that the punches he gave makes him win by experience. Runners can run so many miles to find ways to train better that they eventually need time to rest and relax. A coach, Kate Tenforde from Runcoach, once told me that she wanted me to take a break from running after she helped me train for continuous marathons. I understood with the level of running I was completing and continued my subscription to the service. Since then, I ran numerous marathons and events, communicated with more coaches for training advice, and ran at the gym or outside home with a new outlook on running.

In business world, people can research events nearby and stay informed by reading periodicals in the newspaper or magazines. In racing too, there are magazines such as *Runner's World*, *Women's Running*, and *UltraRunning Magazine* that offer news, training advice, and stories. I subscribe to the *Wall Street Journal*, *Bloomberg Businessweek*, *Fortune*, and *Forbes*, and by knowing my current events,

I can adapt to different reactions with vendors, merchants, customers, and employees daily. If a runner notices they have an ego, they can leave it at the door to not get hurt. A positive image of yourself after a marathon can give you assurance to rest, knowing that the information you read either from promotions for the race or about the community has helped you.

I gain a sense of confidence when in my community shopping and also working because I'm happy to spend and earn my money wisely. Protein bars, shoes, shorts, hats, electrolytes, and treadmills are just a few items that are usually for sale in a running store. Running can improve your health and life expectancy, and in my life, I've been disabled since 1999 through medical conditions that are psychological that made me file for state disability through the state of California. Today, I am working to get through the disability with two jobs, writing, Toastmaster International Clubs, and running when I can.

At one time at the brink of the COVID-19 pandemic, I had four jobs, and when I got gas at the local ARCO gas station, I'd communicate as a friend with a cashier about my progress and activity. Other gas stations such as Costco require memberships and don't need a cashier for service, which is cheaper.

If you run and feel your back ache because of improper form, you can overcome it with your running posture to be upright and slightly tilted forward. The nature and scenery in a race can improve phycological well-being, and with time off a job means you are ready to handle the stressful situations when they arise. Running also reduces stress, anxiety, depression, and tension and allows you time to have adequate sleep, and as an independent contractor for Uber Eats, I need to be mentally alert and get adequate sleep.

A person that lives comfortably with their family is in a place where they are loved, and they can have gratitude toward that. Many times, people create their own families by getting married and having kids, and they live happily in another home and environment. Family living can make you spend more with your parents and siblings and let you have someone that will listen to you. A coach can assist you with the various things such as how many miles you run per day or the types of food to eat, and a parent can listen to your emotions.

This feeling of autonomy can come with earning a higher degree such as an MBA, and relaxation comes as an added benefit that is well deserved for the runner to be able to experience it not just at the gym but in every area they go to. One thing to consider is to be careful while getting your relaxation because you do not want to relax so much that you feel tired behind the wheel. If you carefully adjust your life plan, you can balance work with enough activity and talk to people the way you want without being intrusive or demanding to carry your success to other places.

Since only about 1 percent of the population finishes a marathon, it can make you feel that only 1 percent of the population understands how you feel. In that respect, you can read about how marathoners have a lifestyle that benefits them and how they live. They have essential needs of getting gas, communicating with an attendant, and getting what they have paid for and what they have worked for so they can be their own friend and then be friends with other people.

Since running is free, you can run anywhere and burn calories too. Running with friends can be a way to have someone with same ability as you run with you. While at the starting line of a marathon, there are many elite runners that seem very ready for the race, which you need to be healthy to see and feel. With an overload in training, you can follow the two-day rule or take two days off after an intense run to your weekly program. By fine-tuning your duration for longer runs, you can add a long run in your weekly training plan.

A runner that gets a better time in a marathon than me who trained less than me could have a different lifestyle and intensity at the way they see running. A runner can get a time of 3:30 for the first time they ran a marathon and tell me, and I feel happy for them.

I have trained every day with seventy to one hundred miles a week. Karma is a way to look at this because no matter how hard you train, by the time you finish your run, you'll have the motivation to run more. Your hard work produces actions that can that set you apart. Perhaps, a more novice runner works a type of job that enables them to be on their feet more and earn a fast time. Even if a runner outpaces me, I still feel my experience with about eighty marathons leaves me able to have a benefit conversation with runners that run faster than me that respect my running experience and lifestyle.

Runners perform better if they train for their distance in a race. For example, aim for forty minutes for a 5K, sixty minutes for a 10K, ninety minutes for a half marathon, and two hours for a marathon throughout the week with one day off between workouts for recovery.

I tried a new way of training while working at my job with Ralphs. I did a running workout in the restroom while being a courtesy clerk, and I was able to successfully finish it and see the reactions of others around me as positive as if it was hard for me.

In the real world, runners often interact with people to see a full circle in where they've come with their abilities to feel comfortable as runners and look forward to future races. Every culture has a different way of looking at things and has their own way of living, but in the United States of America, as a productive citizen, you can build your own life and earn your own living. By living with other cultures and carefully noting your own work either by journaling or being careful in situations where you have, you can live life to the fullest.

A person who runs can be a part of a community, have fun, accomplish a goal, and learn work ethic. While running in marathons, there are many business theories that I've studied that I remember, and people cheer for me through pleasant thoughts. I tend to see the course of a run as a manageable challenge. I've seen many courses, and each course has different markers that show me that I am in the right place at the right time. Other motivating factors of running is living healthy with a proper diet and later having time to see how you feel after your run. Knowledge of current events let runners feel in the moment more and more ready for the volunteers handing out water and others trying to get ahead.

This feeling of existence and being alive comes in life when you are at home, work, or outside running. Many people will give you things that you pay for such as food, clothing, gas, shelter, or insurance, and that can be used for your essential priorities.

There can be a time in life when younger people seem to have more influence on you because you might feel a similarity in the person, which is positive. In my experience with younger people either at stores or with customers, there are mixed reaction that can occur, but it is a positive thing to build on those because I can relate to the customer service they give. As a child grows up, goes to school, goes to work, and lives in the real world, that person becomes influenced by the decisions that older people make. Oftentimes a person can see a younger person with an authority that is larger than them to make them motivated. If I make a purchase at a diner and a young person is taking my order as a service, there are factors such as manners that come into play that can influence how I perceive others.

When I am running in a marathon, the city lights, motels, stores, and gas stations often open and close and people come in and out of the stores while law enforcement is often at the sidelines making it a journey. A way to see this as a guiding light is see yourself through each instant on the course as making a push to be more positive and respected in your life.

A runner can reduce stress with good ideas, improve heart health, and help lessen symptoms of depression because it is an aerobic exercise. Running can be good for you in your community because we've evolved to do. A beginner can start to train for at least three days a week, with a longer run on the weekend. After adequate training with running at a conversational pace, you can try to run a 5K or 10K. Resting on your days off can push yourself to feel you know yourself better and see many people want your friendship and take on the possibility of longer runs.

Running can make you live longer, have better sleep, improve immunity, enhance mood, and allow you to read with more passion. After a marathon, my body gets tired, and I need to turn off my computer before bed and rest because of the activity my body went through to emerge as a stronger and happier runner.

In the running brochures that the race produces by press for the runners, it often shows what to expect each mile run in the race, and it makes more sense when I'm running. After a race, it's often best to eat a well-balanced meal, read a periodical or magazine, and have a treat every now and then to unwind and relax. I can process information after running proficiently because of my gratitude in my miles and that my senses are more open to understand the stories better.

Proper training for a run can be a way to relieve your mind of doubt for a race. Training through constant exercise, runs, or by a change in physical activity prepare your mind for the challenges you are about to incur. By avoiding comparing yourself to other runner, you can keep in mind that you accomplished your goals and praise the other person for what they accomplished. In addition to rest and sleeping well, a runner can support others in their training by reading their weekly training summaries. For example, Runcoach has a blog to read from other runners that work hard, and you can support them in their accomplishments. Running as fast and hard as you can on the course can encourage you to perform well with the various obstacles such as the heat, finding restrooms, staying well hydrated, and stretching. The body needs energy to run efficiently and during runs through relaxing your upper body, checking your foot strike, bending your knees, using your arms, and breathing well.

In preparation for a race, I had a talk with a trainer at my former local gym, and I explained to him how much training and exercise I do for each race. He acknowledged my training style and gave me a word of encouragement to eat enough calories after long runs and told me to save my energy for the runs. This helped me to perform better, but if you have the time to train with fueling up on a high carbohydrate and moderate protein meal three to four hours before the race, then you will have energy needed before a longer run. I notice that the more training I do before the race, the more comfortable I become weeks before the race. With a difference in training schedule that can occur because of work, I'm able to still finish a marathon comfortably and stay fueled with electrolytes, water, and snacks during the race. The fastest marathon runners should take at least one week off after a marathon and go for a few short jogs to get back on track and, in two weeks, do light training. After a marathon, nine to ten hours of sleep for a few nights will support recovery, and the usual amount of sleep needed is seven to eight hours.

Strength training exercises two to three sessions per week is a way to prepare your legs to perform well during a marathon, and adding push-ups and pull-ups can help you finish you run. If that is not available to you either because of your work schedule, train your emotional state to deal with the pain.

A runner can build a running resume with their progression over the years starting with high school, and my experience at my gymnasium includes physical, social, and mental performances with best times in distances and mileage. I take time for myself and enjoy the feeling of independence while running. I learn a variety of things in life such as that running and jogging are both form of aerobic exercise that release endorphins, and I try to see my doctor for a checkup before starting a running program. A runner can find a plan called a zone that is effective and includes different types of workouts such as sprinting with varying frequency, duration, and intensity spaced out so you have time to recover.

In Zone 1 jogging, you can run at 50 or 60 percent of your heart rate and maintain control with how fast you can run and how long of a distance you run. The difference of Zone 2 is that you are running at 60 or 70 percent of your heart rate, and Zone 4 is 80 to 90 percent of your heart rate, which is an aerobic or marathon pace for ten to sixty minutes. It is challenging to sustain this rate because you'll feel out of your comfort zone. Your body is adapting itself in the ways that you intended it to, and you can let your body recover, retrain, and prepare better so the next time you are healthy at the starting line of a race.

By being healthy at the starting line, you are at an advantage because you have put months of mileage, talk with friends about your goals, and want to run a new personal record (PR). If you choose unhealthy prerace nutrition, you could feel physically and mentally drained, dizzy, and fall short of your goal race day. By being able to communicate with others before the start of a race, you're grateful for the opportunity and ready to race; you can go out fast and rest later.

You could feel relaxed and calm at the start of the race because you know you've done the work, and you can go out and have fun. Each mile can be a celebration of the hard work you've done to prove that your fit. By the time you get to the last few miles, you can experience a runner high as you are thrilled with your work of effective planning, expert timing, and flexibility.

To help yourself not to get exhausted at the start of a race, you can feel the energy of the other runners near you and keep a safe distance to inspire you. The first few miles of a marathon can be the hardest; your heart pumps blood faster, and your blood vessels deliver more oxygen to your muscles as blood flows to other organs as you run before these organs have fully caught up. There can be some shoves and pushes that are caused by running too close to others or by adjusting yourself to keep your cool, but that is normal. The way to be able to keep a pace is done by slowing down and looking ten feet in front of you, and you can check your breath and breathe through your nose instead of your mouth. Tune into your body and what you feel, and run with your legs straight with your center of gravity over the legs in a stable way.

Runners that are ahead of you often walk at times and let go of their expectations. In a full marathon race, run as fast as you can from start to finish, knowing your own talent and conditioning levels. As you run, find your quickest pace and maintain it by making adjustments to pace on how you feel.

There are times in a race when you can enjoy nature more because you can see the sun at different places and be able to envision where you can find time to rest later. In the United States, people often tell Iranians to have a good day at the nighttime because in Iran it is the daytime when it is nighttime in the United States. Resting at a later time after a race prevents injury and improves running. In a race, the idea of resting later can help you know yourself and the limits of your body to perform better.

The concept of running by time works better if you are on a tight schedule, and running by distance helps you stay motivated. If you plan a thirty-minute run, you can find that it works better than running three to four miles. The inclination that many good things are ahead of you will not ruin your ego of reaching a number of miles. In being able to run at a faster pace, you are able to pick up a new respect for yourself, and it can benefit you in other ways outside of running.

In my training for marathons, I have chosen a pace that works for me or a goal time of about 3:30. It is a formidable goal, but at that time, it's a little bit challenging to achieve. With Runcoach online chats and training, the coaches helped me to choose a goal time such as 3:30 or 3:00, which makes me feel similar to the training of the fastest marathon runners. The fastest runners in the world have been able to get 2:30 or even below two hours in a full marathon, and a goal time that is too fast can also make you feel like you set an unrealistic expectation of yourself.

A realistic goal time can make you more motivated and inspire you to run faster and train better to give you that extra push in your race. There are many ways to set your goal time; one of which is to see your recent marathon time and aim to run twenty minutes faster in your next marathon. In Runcoach training, you can see your projected finish time based on your most recent run. One of the most intelligent ways to train is to ask your coaches training and nutrition questions when you need help to feel more assured for your race. By feeling more assured and prepared, I have more confidence when I'm running and more ability to run at a faster pace. I keep track of my miles running with many platforms such as Runcoach, which lists all my races completed, upcoming races, and lets me manage training preferences to change my schedule. RunSignUp, Strava, Runkeeper, Nike, and Runcoach show my splits too. I write my races along frequency of restroom usage to give my gastrointestinal (GI) doctor a better scope of my overall health.

My pace for recent races has been from twenty minutes per mile to five minutes per mile. When I am taking my Chihuahua for a walk, I'm usually at a mobile pace because I have my dog on a leash and she follows me at a comfortable pace. When I take brisk walks on my own, I can maintain a healthy weight and lose fat and improve muscle endurance. At a gym on a treadmill, there are options at your own discretion to increase pace to about five minutes per mile to feel as the fastest runners do. While running on a course, your body needs to be prepared, and pace can be improved with speed workouts that are comfortable for you. You can run at a pace that seems fast and keep it if you mentally prepare well. Try to build your pace gradually and to avoid injury.

Frequency of training such as running three to five days a week at a relaxed pace is sensible to start. It is important to listen to your body and its signals to adjust accordingly. The world can also bring you success to a point where you feel that after your hard work, you are able to live comfortably and make a living for yourself. You, too, can get to where you want to be in life with long runs and a program for yourself to see that there are no limits in life. The running journey can start with feeling tempo running of ten miles and later determining your rest days.

By acknowledging and lessening common mistakes that occur with runners, such as buying shoes that look good but don't fit or training on pavement when you have a trail run, you can learn from them and move on. When a runner has only one goal in mind such as finishing a marathon, they can often get hurt in the process, but if you have multiple end goals such as getting an extra medal, trying to run a certain pace, or drinking more water, your race will be more elated. Oftentimes age-grade awards are given to the top three of your age group, and while striving toward the top, you grow as you are aiming for higher standards.

A finish line party for a marathon is optional, but often you need to pay a little bit more for before a race and to have VIP finisher party. In this party, you can have special foods, a massage area, and a be in an area that is reserved for certain finishers. The place can let the runner relax and enjoy their experience in a different way, often with music. The San Francisco Marathon offers a finish line party, and in the ultramarathon, there is a finish line area or tent that you can enjoy without paying an extra fee.

If you know your weak areas such as overtraining or picking the wrong training plan, you can put together a training plan to slowly increase pace to run faster. The water stops in a run is a place that a person can hydrate and build energy to continue to run. In the real world, there are many stops including stop signs while driving or challenging customer service situations where you need to call a manager. The challenge can also be while driving to the race when you feel tired and need to pull over to take a walk. Sometimes people arrive late to their race, and if you drove to the race, try to get to the starting line one hour early. But if you're flying, learn to arrive twenty-four hours before the start of the race for your body to recover from the plane.

By running a number of hours in a day and the week, it can look as if you have a lot of other work to finish. The reality of it is that running allows you to see the work that you are about to do as second nature, and that's why so many runners have established careers. It's in the runner's mind that he is able to take in the quickness achieved from runs and maintain their careers to perform well.

Running with a successful training period requires training three days a week, with running at least two days a week for thirty minutes. With all the activities to do in a day, if you plan on a weekend maintenance run for one to two hours, it is an excellent way to get some perspective on your abilities. A runner can watch television, listen to the news on radio, or listen to people at work, then be able to take in the benefits they got from running and eating healthy.

Age-grade running is a statistical attempt to measure the comparative strength of a performance for an athlete of a certain age, and a runner who's fifty and runs a 5K in twenty minutes is more impressive than a twenty-year-old runner who runs it in eighteen minutes.

The runners find many ways to experience joy with others, and I give credit to myself for my accomplishments. The running etiquette on the road is usually to run facing traffic with your head up, wear reflective clothing, and obey the traffic rules. I also run with my fist or hands going back and forth in a manner that is comfortable. The more comfortable you get with your style, the more you can adjust it when needed. The joy comes in instances when you can feel a runner high, happiness, or a natural bliss that may be when you are in control of your body and mind as you can process personal struggles and make creative ideas.

In marathons, there is a state of running where you have long distances that can either be flat or on hills. Most running is on flat surfaces, and running on hills uses your energy to build your endurance, speed, and power to make you faster. Downhill running on a course strengthens your bones and muscles but stresses your joints and muscles. Happiness and smiling through running can be maintained with plenty of exercise, being grateful, and breathing deeply to find a balance in areas of your life that you did not see before. Also, by fine-tuning your daily habits to be more positive, you can gradually make lasting change to run various distances with joy.

The way to gain a better experience with hill running is to have consistency behind you and to lean into the hill. Most of my virtual runs start and end on a hill, and you are keeping a fast pace and increasing intensity through hills. Most times in running a course or just outside your home, you'll find a constant pace and won't feel a need to slow down. Often, hills make up 15 percent of your run, and oftentimes my finishing pace on hills can be five minutes above my average pace because the body's energy levels are kept strong when you tell yourself you are trying your hardest to finish strong.

Runners can proceed beyond a limit to be ahead of others in many ways such as by starting at the front of a course. An athlete keeps themselves more fit than a sedentary person who watches television all day. In the journey of finding a level of comfort and avoiding the sedentary lifestyle, try to walk for five minutes every two hours and find the aspects of your life that you need help to adjust accordingly.

The normal productive citizen in today's society contributes to their nation by being productive and can be employees and people from many professions. The people who exercise every day that try hard for their body to be in shape or healthier than their previous lifestyle can be productive. It can be years before feeling satisfied with your body, but if you love yourself as your neighbor, you can make your goal feasible. At times, I ran twenty miles a day for several days a week, and I found that by setting time aside to run was more of a passion and joy than a chore. In my quest for happiness, the natural movements of my body can release endorphins to release stressors.

The time you've spent through a course of a race with getting an end result and finishing indeed makes you more familiar to know how to manage your time and be well prepared. The ability to say to yourself that you can perform with searching harder for a plan is essential because you can get to a point where you need to have a system of support when possible. There are places that can seem more familiar in a course especially if you've run it before. In the long run, it helps to know where you are going, and by knowing where to run and where the aid stations are, you can have a more successful race. The experience of running brings a sense of calmness that you can see when you feel the energy.

Running helps the spirit to show your determination and focus and reminds us of our goal to go beyond former limits. Spiritual runners can live and cohabit with the sport to run with the goal of meditation. Some app such as Fitbit, Strava, and Runcoach have online tools that can give you special awards or badges as an ongoing symbol of your achievement. For example, one time, I earned a Satellite badge with Fitbit with thirty-five thousand lifetime floors. It had an interesting design, and the badge can be shared too.

Certain marathon offers runners a badge through the race website or an app called RTRT.me for completing a marathon or a number of miles and be downloaded and printed as a special rememberable experience for your work done. The San Francisco Marathon, for example, gave me a downloadable badge after finishing the marathon and ultramarathon. Many law enforcements officers wear badges ranging from the police, firefighters, to Homeland Security officials in airport that can show pride in their careers for their particular profession. A marathon badge lets runner know he can go through similar obstacles on a course finding a way through the roads, volunteers, and officials to complete a race within a finish time.

A similarity of careers of hard-working officials with badges to a runner can be that a runner achieves a similar feeling of autonomy and accomplishment after their race and their badges can be kept for a lifetime.

In most races, there are a variety of opportunities for discounts given when registering for the current or future races. It could seem to be a lot of expenses to still pay at the expo since you feel that you have prepared well for your race, but now you have to make decisions about the next race to register for, but this is a matter of preference with your decision.

In addition to earning medals and online badges for my running efforts, there have also been ways that the running clubs have assisted me to show appreciation for some of my running feats. Recently I was recognized with seven hundred miles stepped badge by Runcoach, where the coach gave me an offer later to buy Garmin gear at a discounted price. The main idea is that however you train and perform, you will later be in a place of reality or a race that you trained for where you are connecting or communicating with other people at a sentimental level. The idea of being able to improve yourself and make the reaches necessary can give you your own edge or a distinct feature that you can now enjoy.

The race expo atmosphere is usually a thrilling environment to participate in because there are many vendors giving away free items, samples to try, and many runners visiting booths to pick up their bib number and shirts. To make the most out the expo, spend less than one hour there, buy merchandise if needed, sign up for drawings, get massages, or even get a chiropractic exam. The vendors often wear marathon expo badges with their names that let you know they are there for you to answer your questions and offer merchandise. It can be a glimpse of how the race will go itself, but most of the time, they will wish you good luck in the race. The customer service skills of people I've met at the gym and work and other places lets me see how the mindset and professionalism of vendors are when they politely try to help me with the race the next day.

The website of the race often has designs such as palm trees that show a theme of the run, and you can view the trees and course, its sponsors, race information, and know what to expect during the event. For example, the Surf City Marathon is a race in Huntington Beach and near the ocean with many palm trees on the side that make the roads look beautiful. The palm trees in a course are similar to the ones seen in various neighborhoods throughout Los Angeles.

When I worked as an account manager at Elite Development Enterprises, I was in many neighborhoods in Los Angeles that had rows of palm trees, and at my local gym, there are palm trees outside. The correlation is that when training and later running a marathon, there are usually no clear-cut ways to know what the course will bring, except the fact that you are given guidelines. The reason that you made it to the run with other runners similar to yourself shows you've prepared well and are ready to make it to the starting line successfully.

The experience of getting to a race and finding parking can be interesting and changes with more and more preparation. If you print out a map and use it as a backup to your GPS on your phone or in your car, you should find the way. In the first part of the day, it takes time to wake up in time and do everything necessary to leave your home or hotel to get to the race on time. If I wake up at 1:00 a.m. or 2:00 a.m., it's often hard work from my normal routine to prepare to drive a few hours to a race because even the newspaper has not made it to the driveway. You have spent a lot of time showering, going online, or eating breakfast. It is important to try to save your energy so you don't get tired with countless other things needed to have a successful day and race.

In eating a healthy meal before a race, it is often better to skip milk because it can make your stomach a little uneasy during your run. I used to set aside protein bars and log them into my Fitbit tracker to save time and experience a pleasurable feeling during the race. Often, I added ten to thirty bars at a time before a race, and my app almost always said I was over target with the number of calories consumed versus absorbed until I finished my race.

Recently, I cut the number of protein bars down to two or none at all. By the time comes to the twentieth or twenty-sixth mile comes, my tracker showed me that I haven't eaten enough calories and I'd need to eat more to keep my body in balance after a marathon. You can get ready a lot quicker in the morning of a marathon than a usual day because at the race expo, the vendors and race staff try to support you for your race to skip a lot of the guesswork to be prepared to take on each challenge in a different way.

The experience of getting safely to the parking lot of a race can be a task worth preparing for because you want to have enough energy before, during, and after the race. In a race, the organizers have a system to everything—from parking, the expo, the race itself, and music played after the finish line—for the organizers to prepare for. All of these can be seen on the website of the race itself because you are able to navigate through the event pages.

As a public speaker, I have been able to shape my speaking skills through a Toastmasters International speaking club where I have given a number of speeches on marathon running and the experience of running itself.

Running gives you an outlook of purpose and openness to new experiences to find time to attend. It also gives you calmness, flexibility, mobility, strength, and social skills because of the interactions that come from a long-distance run. The social ability to maintain confidence in my speaking skills about my achievements in running give me autonomy in my life. By participating in Toastmaster International groups as a member of two clubs, The Health and Wellness Toastmasters and Top Sales, I'm improving public speaking skills where I've talked numerously about running marathons to the public.

As member of Toastmasters International, I got to higher positions such as the vice president of Public Relations and the club coach, and I'm a two-time area director today, presently with Division D1. This position is an executive position that allows me to channel information among the clubs and division and district leadership. I'm in charge of six local clubs and guide them to meet the mission of helping members grow. While running virtual runs, I can communicate with Toastmasters through Zoom and maintain an adequate speed, giving me the ability to multitask. Many professional runners make records, and others follow and make their own goals based on what they believe they can achieve.

I have given many running speeches that the members of my Health and Wellness Toastmasters club got tired of hearing, and I gradually changed my speeches to include a variety of other interesting topics such as Chihuahuas. For example, I have given a speech about various marathons on a PowerPoint presentation that had many slides explaining many marathons along with the website addresses and pictures of medals, runners, and the race itself.

The Lexus LaceUp Running Series had events such as the Ventura Marathon, Palos Verdes Half Marathon, Riverside Half Marathon, and Orange County Marathon, and the series now has been discontinued in 2022.

Another speech that I've done was regarding the 2019 San Francisco Ultramarathon, which is what got me to go back to being a member of Toastmasters International. The speech included explaining my Toastmasters' fundraising event, which was a success for me because many members donated money to me to make my trip feasible. I found that the fees needed to run the race were rather high or about $400 for the race itself and another $400 for the hotel and airline. Also, food expenses can run high during a trip, which made me decide my second fundraising event for the San Francisco Marathon. I handed out various brochures and fliers for the event at the meeting and got a positive response, which made me feel well.

The first lap of the course was explained to me that it started in reverse with various crowds outside at 12:00 a.m. waiting to see a movie and different landmarks such as the Golden Gate Bridge were presented. The challenging part of the race for me was explained, which was getting lost and rerouted and needing to find the correct places to use the restrooms. With feedback from the director himself, Michael Li, who called me after the race discussing my experience, it made me more prepared, listening more to the prerace talk and prepare better the next race. Now I know to ask the volunteer cyclists to cut off the locks for the porta potties ahead of time and how to ask for assistance for medical items by telephone while on course.

The journey of running race successfully and later looking back is ongoing where you can learn how to pick up some pieces to improve. The more a person can look forward and not feel afraid that someone behind them is catching up, the better. A runner that no longer runs to win is afraid of losing and look back to make sure you have a comfortable distance with them on the race. Oftentimes, I can reflect on looking backward to ask runners if I'm running in the right direction and can tell me which way to go, or they could be running another distance such as a half marathon and not know what to tell me.

With the running world, I have made it to several clubs that put me in a place of recognition for achievement. After ten consecutive years of running in the full Long Beach Marathon, there was a Lighthouse Park bench that my name and other eligible members' name had been enshrined to the plaque on the 2019 Run of Fame Bench in Lighthouse Park. Many of the other runners ran consecutive half marathons to achieve the feat, and it was first planned to be set somewhere in Long Beach. I brought my parents with me to the race expo, and the plaque was revealed to the Beach Bum members and me. It was an exciting feeling to be with a select group of runners. Beach Bum members also get special discounts to future events sponsored by Shock Top and VIP Race Weekend Experience, and there is a Shock Top Beach Bum members-only area adjacent to the beer garden at the finish line.

The running journey can also bring you a new perspective on how you see your peers or how younger generations perceive you and interact with you. You can often look and feel younger than your age and see your family and others around you also grow in life. In efforts to connect more with my peers, I joined a group of people called Project Return Peer Support Network or Project Peer to Peer Return, which was a distinctive mental health nonprofit organization where staff use their experience to serve others with mental challenges. I met with a group of members and a facilitator that took time to recognize each other with bowling or a three-mile walk at Wilson Park in Torrance, which was harder for me to attend to because of my work schedule. The idea was to connect with people older than you so you could return to the point of life where you feel more comfortable interacting with them.

The idea of meeting people in the neighborhood where you live is also something that is beneficial to you and your neighbor because you feel good when you introduce yourself. There is the saying that you should love your neighbor or to do unto others as you will do to yourself. The way a runner is able to experience a marathon and have a pleasant and exciting run can be similar to someone going to a town that they have not been in before who look at the maps to see the landmarks they can visit and see. For example, in the San

Francisco Marathon expo, oftentimes a map of the city is given to help the runner know the city areas better, and it has helped me after checking into my hotel to find places to go in the city including where to go to walk to the expo.

In racing and believing in yourself, you have an idea that your finish time will be fine, as long as you run at your own steady pace with courage and endurance. The courage to step up your run comes from within at times to get to the finish and receive your medal. Positive feedback from seeing other runners and pacers or volunteers affiliated with the marathon can give kind words to encourage you, and you can work and build from their feedback.

Runners and volunteers can be saying things to you such as "I like it, keep it up" or "Good job" that make you believe that the marathon journey is still being written because you are getting to conquer your goals. There are still records to break, achievements that have not been set, and new theories to be written about ways to run faster. Also, marathons can continue to improve with new courses, more nutrition on the course, new sponsors, and new challenges to write to continue the history of how a marathon evolves. In the events that led you to getting to your race, there have been many current events in the city, promotions, and information to absorb that can help you be able to stay present and knowledgeable for your run.

The journey of learning more about yourself and healthier eating habits as a runner can lead you to make better choices in almost all aspects of your life because you feel that you know yourself better and can eat better. For example, food such as cheeseburgers and french fries don't make you feel strong when running. Later try to lessen those foods and substitute them with a grilled chicken sandwich and fruits and see how you feel.

When you are running, you can put your body to the test to see if your pace improves and then make adjustments to your diet for improved performance of your future runs. By listening to your body while running, you can know not only to avoid injury, but you can also improve your average running speed and know when to take out protein bars if you relied on them.

When a person walks their dogs in a neighborhood, it is necessary to clean up their waste with a bag because neighbors don't want to clean others' waste. When a person sets out to run a race, it also is necessary to clean up your own waste and to toss or recycle the cups of water and electrolytes in nearby bins, use the porta potties when needed, and discard your trash or food wrappers in nearby bins. Oftentimes a volunteer will not clean up your trash if they feel that you just threw it on the ground. It is necessary to be careful, considerate, and mindful to the volunteers so you have the confidence to race positively. If you feel that you could have conducted communication with a volunteer better such as by answering their question more politely, there is no need to feel tension because you're running and have the assurance of many other volunteers ahead of you.

Three to four days a week of time aside to run can be sufficient to keep your body well-tuned, but if you don't have the time to train to run, walking a fifteen-minute mile can help you sustain a longer run. Focus on good interactions, feedback, and the strength of other runners to improve your mental health instead of recalling bad running experiences you've had.

There are some good things to consider while running such as the pleasant memories of people you have worked with that can give you more of an edge and mental focus. Your likes and dislikes with food and customer service have a lasting effect on your present time, and if remember yourself and your environment in your stronger runs, your focus will develop. There are many chefs that make oven-fresh pizza by making the dough, rolling it, baking it in the oven with cheese, marinara sauce, and toppings to be enjoyed; but when consumed in moderation and prepared in wholesome ways, it can be an excellent food for runners.

A business owner who opens their store to make pizza can get it to the customer either by pickup or delivery, and runners can see a learning process because if they choose whole-wheat pizza after their run with vegetables, they can feed their bodies well instead of eating pizza twelve hours before their run.

I had a job delivering pizza at an appetizer restaurant when I was seventeen years old, and when I was seven, I visited Italy with my parents and ate pizza in a restaurant. Talking with my parents makes me feel that pizza isn't balanced well and is suboptimal for athletes. I visited many pizza restaurants while in middle school in the Palos Verdes with family, and I got to see Italian culture and the Italian love of family. Pizza is a food that can make you lose energy and feel lethargic, and it can add on pounds if you don't exercise it off. If you are a healthy runner, you can include pizza or a large meal and run four hours later and be in good shape.

With the types of food and choices that runners make, there are times your experience on the course can sense the reasons you visited so many pizza and fast choices for restaurants. Pizza has been popular in my life after my MBA graduation ceremony at California State University Dominguez Hills. My mom and her friends took pictures of me near a pizza vendor on campus called Three Brothers Pizza, and with all of the essays, business theories, and research papers written, the booth had meaning to me as a graduate with advanced degree taking a picture and smiling.

Pizza first came into my life after I went BMX biking with my childhood friends where we would always eat pizza, usually from Domino's, to celebrate the time we had burning calories. Pizza is also given to runners after the Orange County Marathon in a special finish line area. I seemed to be the only one who would take off the cheese to save calories.

As the saying goes, "Junk in, junk out," if you eat healthy, you will feel healthy. If you eat unhealthily, you will feel unhealthy and possibly feel unhealthy racing. In choosing to eat healthy, you fuel your body the right way with an easily digested meal or snack before a run. When it comes to fast food, unhealthy selections can lead to a drop in performance. Chicken and fish can be healthy choice in restaurants if it's baked, grilled, broiled, or skinless; but at the typical fast-food place, most choices come deep fried or breaded with lots of mayonnaise that has saturated or unhealthy fat. If more fast-food places adopt healthier menus to include choices of pasta with ground turkey or with fish, more people would avoid high sugar junk food, which makes you fatigued.

Oftentimes marathoners can eat fast food because it can be a fuel for a long race and the sugar can convert to energy. One can look like a bodybuilder in a gym or a marathon runner surrounded by a number of people who eat the calories they need and burn them off later.

In addition to eating healthy, a runner can find hobbies such as playing Jenga, bowling, watching movies, going to sporting games, collecting coins, or reading magazines—all of which I've enjoyed. For most races that are over three hours of drive away, I find it easier to reserve a hotel room to save energy, shower after the race, and watch television instead of driving my way to race because there's also time for some hobbies such as watching a movie in a movie theater.

All of these factors can influence your performance with runners and your community because after you shower, you'll feel cleaner once you arrive home. If you see yourself successful after finishing a race, that is excellent. When should you take in your accomplishment? After you work at your job. Months or years after the race? It's best to recognize your achievement after you cross the finish line, after you get your medal, or after you get your finisher certificate or order photos to have peace of mind and view your accomplishment.

Runners start their race by registering first, later successfully participating, and sometime later seeing that your money was spent well in community marathons. Some virtual marathons can cost about $20 while smaller marathons cost about $120, and small big-city marathons are near $300. There is prize money for top finishers that can be as high as $150,000. Getting the understanding of society where you live by learning of community events can motivate you to be more involved. In the community, after you are rested and recovered, you can feel a push in the right direction to pick up where you left off at an earlier point in life. If you had a problem with public speaking or were shy socially, you can later get through the insecurities by talking in public about the things that made you start running.

When I register for a race, I purchase the race registration from the merchant or online and later run the race and earn a prize or medal. When I talk to a merchant at a restaurant or other store with my job at Uber Eats, I see that they are preparing food for a customer that I will deliver to, and there is distance that I must drive to complete my delivery and earn money merchant to settle. When registering for a marathon, oftentimes the vendor or merchant can be in another state or far off the city. The fact that you are the one who paid for it and you are still in the same place is one thing, but as a runner, you'll travel to the race area and complete the race mile after mile. The experience of getting what you want in life can be a positive one if you feel happy to get what you paid for and earn a prize such an age division award in a marathon.

The ability to keep your head up, hands loose, arms close to you, engage your core, and gaze forward while running can help you keep better running form. Social distancing of six feet while running and wearing a mask and gloves can help you run in modern times. The changes in form such as avoiding tilting your head down and slumping your shoulders can be worked on by holding your shoulders back and lifting your head to lessen strain on your back. In being able to work and learn, you can build your running skills and continue to grow versus if you are running with no job and fall.

The way to keep yourself nourished for a run can start very early in the day or at breakfast. Prior to a race or event, you will see various marathon event staff assisting runners to go to an area inside of the expo. These event staff are often full of energy and only let runners in that paid extra for the race or are VIP members, which can be enough fuel for yourself at the later parts of the race when other staff help runners after the event because you have finished.

There have also been many offers given to me to be an ambassador for a race but were not taken because I'd rather run and enjoy the race without the added responsibilities. In being an ambassador, there are often qualifications needed such as in San Francisco, you would need to be an experienced runner with significant social media presence such as five hundred Instagram followers, ties to the racing community, and participate in community outreach. Often, the ambassador undertakes to represent and promote the race for certain benefit or perks such as discounts to future events.

The marathon experience can be seen by yourself as a journey to better know who you are and your capabilities because as you see your previous race results, you can plan to do better. Once you find your capabilities and your projected time of finishing, you can plan for your race by letting the event staff know your time from last year's run to qualify for a corral. For example, in the 2022 Los Angeles Marathon, in a seeded corral, you are put in a special group of the fastest 7,300 runners based on previous marathon finish times. I have started in corrals way at the front named A when my corral would actually start at D. This is always a positive because you can start the race with the fastest runners who have a projected target finish of about 3:30. In doing this, you are putting yourself at the front of the race, at your own discretion, and it has been my choice in the majority of marathons to go to the front of the pack to often run twenty minutes faster.

The corral starts are wave starts for bigger races to reduce cramming so the groups run in a similar pace. The faster runners won't get too close to each other and also leave room for the slower runners when they can. The way to build yourself as a runner is similar to someone who is bodybuilding, but bodybuilders usually don't run marathons. There is the body itself, and later you as a runner are getting ready to run by dressing in shirts, shorts, socks, shoes, a fanny pack, a bib number, and anything else that is needed; but at the end of the race, you will get a pretty medal to hang around your neck. In perspective, a bodybuilder visits a gymnasium and uses powder if necessary for lifts, wears a weight belt if needed, has shorts, a shirt, socks, shoes, a fanny pack, gloves, and anything else needed. The difference is that the bodybuilder does not usually get a medal after he is done lifting and can't maintain a pace as a marathoner does, but he can enjoy his time after lifting weights that are mental in comfort by letting his aggression go by communicating that he is done. A weight lifter can move about so much in the gym that by the time he is done, he is as exhausted as a marathon runner but still in the gym.

The ability to run throughout a race can give you a sense of discipline. The discipline last longer for you after your run to incorporate into other areas of your life. For example, if running relieves stress and anxiety or even muscle pain as you run, it will help you later in your daily life to continue to relieve pain. The same goes for when you are running or exercising. The more effort you put in, the more tired you will feel, but later in the day, you will feel much better after your body has recovered. The rest after runs is a way that your body naturally becomes stronger. The physical effort you put in through running lets you feel more energized later, and you'll have the ability to rest longer or even get better sleep.

There have been times when I felt I would not be running as much, but those feelings left, and I began to run even more. The race series called Series Runner features runs or races all throughout the United States, and with the challenge, you can complete an ultra, full, or half marathon within the series. If the race has a virtual option, you can get credit for it in the challenge running virtually instead of having to travel because you can run up to 50 percent of your runs virtually while qualifying for the challenge. The Series Runner Challenge is meant to be simple; you are the architect that can travel, run, interact with people, and find areas in life to excel in. In 2020, all runs could be run virtually, and I completed about twenty marathons for the twenty-race series medal.

The Series Runner Challenge had something that was not typical for me to see, which was races out of the state of California, including Texas, Pacific Northwest, Utah, Colorado, Arizona, Nevada, Oregon, and Washington, which makes it enjoyable to have a large selection of races to choose from that are reputable.

In my first Series Runner medal, I completed the challenge with a mix of physical races that included local races in Southern California. The way a runner can stay motivated year-round is to have an achievement plan to follow for success. The way to run and enjoy your race continues long after you're finish to the present moment. From starting to run, running, finishing, and later planning your next event, the runner is able to have many opportunities to learn how to run smarter the next time from experience. In addition to getting a medal, you are preparing yourself to be stronger and in a better place than where you were earlier.

In me accomplishing twenty races or twenty-one for the Series Runner Challenge, I lost access to my local gym because of the shutdown for COVID-19. In my own mind, I knew I had a lot of potential with all my training and that there should be ways to show it. In life's reality, how you feel and think toward goals eventually pays off if you find the proper way to put it forth. In running over twenty races in three weeks, some of the doctors I saw wanted me to take it differently. They told me to slow it down because they did not want me to get injured, which was fine, but I intended to finish the 2020 Series Runner Challenge on my own pace.

To see my story for the Series Runner running series that I've completed, I was asked by a race administrator as to what my motivation was to complete a twenty-race challenge. My answer was that by giving the time to complete races on my own, I was able to still work with two jobs—one at Ralphs and the other as a delivery driver—and have the time to run races on my own. I had a pleasant experience training for these runs with proper diet and an exercise schedule given to me by a Future app from 24 Hour Fitness and Runcoach that has workouts set for me every day to stay fit and run a faster pace throughout the races.

I was also in the process of writing my current book, *The Running Journey*, and was motivated to see my story be shown in an email by Series Runner as a "Runner that Pushes through COVID-19."

As a resident of Rancho Palos Verdes, I started running at the age of ten in the Catalina Island, running 10K with my father. Now I run because it gives me a sense of comfort and the ability to feel healthy. One of my goals was that I lost one hundred pounds since 2009, and I kept it off through consistently exercising and running. Some inspiration to me is seeing past Olympians that were marathon runners and my father who was an avid cyclist. It did not seem possible for me to finish the twenty-race Series Runner Challenge this year, but I did it in three weeks. It was five-state run in three weeks virtually, and now I have the medals hanging in my room.

A virtual run has many benefits that a physical run does not have such as being able to run a new course every time you run. In 2020, when I set out to run twenty races for the Series Runner

Challenge, I ran a different course each and every race. For example, one race I would run to Redondo Beach and witness many beach-going people enjoy their day at the beach by either sunbathing, playing volleyball, eating food, bodyboarding, surfing, skateboarding, riding a bike, walking, running, roller-skating, or even flying in a kitelike machine. The way to run by the beach is always an amazing experience because you have many lifeguards protecting the beach, many emergency vehicles making the beach safe, and many things to do such as exploring all the options that beachgoers have while running on a beach, including FindABeach app.

My experience with running shows me that these challenges are appealing because I ran nearly 400 miles in one month in 2021, which was a very active month, and I also completed the 2021 Series Runner Challenge for the 500-mile run medal or a total of 524 miles run. When it comes to reading about the races that are more selective, it can give you a glimpse of how the rich and famous enjoy their lifestyles. For example, oftentimes the rich and famous are able to have their lives set to a point of luxury, but a gifted runner can also experience similar happiness as does the top 1 percent of the richest people because the neighborhoods that the rich people live in are accessible by the experience the runners have. When you search to come out of a situation where only 1 percent of the population has also done, you are able to find that truth in the statistic that only 1 percent of the population can run a marathon.

Running as a hobby, sport, or other enjoyment in your life can make you feel satisfied with your goals. The body and mind connect, and you can feel stimulated to be on the right path and track. The running with well-being and stability is something you can improve upon daily by journaling, exercising, reading, and working. Setting a goal to run has helped me most because I made time and set attainable goals with races.

The goal of 500 miles for the 2021 Series Runner Challenge a lot of races that I registered for either virtually or in person. I finished the challenge with 524 miles and was one of the top earners of the challenge. Most of the races I chose at the start of the year were virtual, and I had about 400 miles by May because I didn't know the challenge rules. The 2021 Series Runner Challenge has changed its rules, and I wasn't aware that physical races must be run to get the challenge medal.

It was a little shock for me at first to see that by running 400 miles I wouldn't get any type of challenge medal and I would have to match my physical miles with virtual miles to get the medal. Today, I am able to travel comfortably within California and the various regions to qualify for the challenge medal at the end of the year. By looking at the near 400-mile run virtually, I had the confidence that I would be able to use at least 250 miles virtually and actually go to other races in person and have some fun. I saw how the challenge rules changed; and with patience, staying safe while traveling, and keeping a good relationship with family, friends, and coworkers, I made the challenge possible.

I made the adjustment calmly and smoothly to get back to the challenge rules. I spoke with the CEO through emails and found that I was able to run any race and any distance to get the challenge medal, but my miles must be an equal mix. After I learned the rules, I found that I had to have an equal mix of virtual and physical miles to get five hundred miles.

I enjoyed signing up for virtual runs because of the comfort of choosing a start time and by having accessibility of roads to run in. I also decided when to submit my results. My preference was to run a race closer to home rather than paying fees to travel to a race because it can be expensive. I enjoy actually going to a physical race more today because I communicate with other runners and have the pleasure of seeing a beautiful course. A completed challenge can help you choose smarter from the various races to register for online.

My goal of getting five hundred miles for the Series Runner Challenge in 2021 was a goal that I had all year long, and I was very happy to get the confirmation of my accomplishment from the CEO and rewards department at Series Runner. The feeling of getting my medal in the mail in March of 2022 was just as I expected because of the size of the medal, and there was a delay in sending out medals because of a factory shutdown. In 2022, the Series Runner challenge seems attainable again for me, and by taking six weeks off extraneous activity due to a surgery, I feel like I can give my body a well-needed rest.

By running a full or half marathon virtually, I felt an ability to conquer a lot of my fears of running such as how much distance I comfortably run. My pace ranged from about nine minutes up to about eighteen minutes, and it improved when my body felt recovered after longer runs. I had a time where my shin was swollen for a few days, and it caused me to run slower, but I was able to recover quickly by being able to jog at a pace that worked for me. I was able to walk the pain away. My ability to see how I was capable of making myself be able to run many events back-to-back was a little bit of a change from running a marathon every few months while training several hours a day at the gym. By running twenty races in three weeks, my body needed more rest. But since I felt up to complete the challenge quickly, so I did.

A change comes from feeling I'm able to complete more races in a shorter period of time than by spacing out seven races throughout the whole year. Often a race has advertising and logos set for the upcoming run one year in advance and can change to let a runner feel the energy in the run to have a pleasant time. The fun part of the journey is seeing the effort that a runner puts into their run and later being able to run with more determination that was set with virtual run. The virtual run basically means that a runner can run a race without actually traveling to a course, but instead they run the race on their own time or anywhere they please and track the time on their watch to later send to the race for their medal.

Many times, the experience of running a virtual marathon by the beach is similar to an actual in-person marathon by the beach. Most beaches open and close their restrooms at a certain time, and it can be important to time your virtual marathon well enough so that by the time you'll finish, the restrooms will not be closed. The beautiful scenery at the beach leaves you with many safe activities to partake in, which are fun if you follow the rules of the beach. Every day the lifeguards write new conditions for beachgoers to see such as the tide, sunset, and surf conditions that lets the beachgoers. Being able to use the restrooms properly during a run or virtual run can make you more disciplined to feel better when you need to go. The more you focus on your running instead of using each restroom, the better you'll feel throughout your race. The ability of the body to take a liking of the athletic world is exciting, and the natural human feeling to improve your racing style is remarkable.

There are many running trails in Palos Verdes that are that are beautiful that also have equestrian access for horses. I've ran the surface streets in Palos Verdes or near Palos Verdes Drive North, which has many paths and trails for walkers and runners. Many of the trails were often closed, but the experience of Palos Verdes trails is exciting because the city once hosted the Palos Verdes Marathon. The reason that the trails are fun is that they are called as reserves such as the Ocean Trails Reserve, Portuguese Bend Reserve, Palos Verdes Bluff Trail, and Forrestal Nature Reserve. The trails go all throughout the city, bringing excitement to run without traveling to another state or city. The runs throughout Rancho Palos Verdes, Rolling Hills Estates, Rolling Hills, Palos Verdes Estates, and neighboring cities are sensational because of the various high-class businesses, churches, and neighboring residential areas.

The difference between a physical or in-person race to a virtual race is something that more runners should experience because if you were used to just running races in person, many would feel like they wouldn't make the change to a virtual race. The change can let a runner see the difference. An in-person race is a guided course that has volunteers without many options. A runner can feel much better once they are able to make the change to a virtual race because they can have the option of postponing the race to another day in the same time frame.

In today's running world, there have been many stoppages of major races due to the COVID-19 pandemic. Today, it's not known if the races that were shut down due to COVID-19 pandemic will continue to be virtual or if they will open up to the public again.

I've looked forward to many races with Series Runner that were canceled until the following year, and the story about me pushing through COVID-19 has made me run more since the start of the pandemic. There are many runners that are just as satisfied with running a race virtually because they can run more flexibly and are able to still get a finisher's medal, T-shirt, and other swag that is sent out. My motivation is higher than ever to complete races in a faster time, and a marathon that takes me four hours on a course today can take me up to seven hours if I run virtually and at a slower pace.

The difference in virtual racing that inspires me the most is the feeling of calmness knowing that I can create my own course and enjoy a 26.2-mile run with my own scenic route and at my own time. The various beaches in Southern California made me learn about how the real world operates and how the public lives with others in various cities. For example, it is possible to run a virtual race for a Series Runner event and later in an in-person race, but you can only get credit for one event since that would make it easy for runners to double up on miles.

By running virtually, there is a possibility that you will place much higher than you would in the physical race or with other races. By placing first place in some of my virtual races, I received age division awards and finisher's certificates and special medals that showed me as first place. It is an outstanding feeling to place first, it can be done with glory without exhausting yourself. Similar to the LaceUp running events where the runners placed first, second, or third and were given an award, I met some of them, and now I feel the enjoyment that they felt by placing first in my division and receiving an award.

The organizers plan their online running events well as many runners decide they want to stay because of COVID-19 and race virtually instead of in person. This allows runners to have an optimistic outlook to their health and the health of others in the races they've registered for and to prepare and train differently. In most races, the website tells you about the virtual option if you click on frequently asked questions, the registration page, or virtual page, and most questions are answered to let the runner plan ahead. By inspecting and studying the race websites before the race, it shows me how to construct a feasible training plan by seeing the course and knowing what to expect.

The different websites let the runner believe they can win and conquer the course and be eligible for the race's prizes and register for the event in the future again.

Keeping awake in the day varies from person to person depending on their lifestyle, and I move around more, and I learned that the aerobic exercise of running causes the brain to discharge endorphins that keep me awake. When it comes the time to sleep, perceptions can differ as to how much sleep you need. Now I try to get eight to nine hours of sleep before and after a marathon and enjoy my day and night with time to wind down before bed.

I learned that races are not as difficult as they appear online because once you get to a course and run, you'll see that you can have fun. In running many virtual races near my home, the races have designed their events for runners to view landmarks and places that they haven't seen or experienced. My idea of setting a faster pace for a race is an admirable goal, but I try to run with a consistent pace and try not to start out too fast and speed up later.

Pace from start to finish can be improved with your outlook, productivity, and change in physical activity. In my journey of running nearly twenty races in three weeks for Series Runner, I built my confidence through keeping a fast pace throughout the whole race. Other times my pace could range from nine minutes eighteen because of foot pain, but during the first seventeen miles, my pace ran at twelve minutes per mile and later at seventeen minutes per mile because I often finished on a hill.

I worked as a Postmates courier before the company was bought by Uber Eats, and I learned to go to a business or restaurant and communicate with merchants to pick up food for a customer and deliver it safely.

A runner improves pace by taking it easier on your body with hard days to push more on easy days because you trust your body. If you work at a corporate business, you might enjoy the office setting in a cubicle or having various businesses close to your office. I've had the experience of being in a cubicle and also in a corporate office, and the activity of sitting on my desk working on my computer seemed to help me participate and interest me to learn more about running.

There are many ways runners improve their mental focus for races such as becoming more involved in their environment by appreciating nature to see that they shouldn't take the beauty for granted. The way that I am able to focus on my surroundings helps me feel more self-ful-filled. I separate my thoughts from pain and let my body flow to run and think away from a cramp. When a stranger enters a strange land, they can feel that they need to work harder to feel adjusted to their environment. As with the stories of many rock and roll bands such as one of my previous favorites, Iron Maiden, a person can be in a setting where they come from another planet to Earth to see themselves in a whole different way to work harder to fit in.

Today, the band's front man, Bruce Dickinson, has been fea-tured on *Forbes* as an airplane pilot and feels the stage lets him see his fans more and continues to make new albums. When a runner is on a course of a marathon or even a virtual marathon, the road is clear and open and many cars are parked on both sides. The sun and heat can cause your body temperature to rise, and the sweat produces water loss from the blood and cause dehydration.

In a dental office visit, you often need to fill out paperwork so the doctor is comfortable to perform your dental work, and you don't want to pay too much for a visit even if you have insurance because the doctor might not do the job right.

A runner on a new course can focus on thinking of things that are positive such as in my life, my father's success with his own busi-ness as a certified public accountant (CPA) and being a professor of accounting at California State University Dominguez Hills often kept me with clarity because I learned as I worked with him. A run-ner can have more comfort and fun in a race than they would in daily life with shopping, dining, or visiting new places as there are always new people to meet. The journey of running a race on hard roads or pavement can be softer or easier on your body than sidewalks. In running on the sidewalk, it can be safer to avoid traffic, and a small part of my virtual runs is on the sidewalk because I choose to run near the roads and against traffic. The announcer for a race prepares the runners with a greeting, opening announcement, national anthem, and encouragements in daily life to enjoy the pleasant things ahead and after the finish line.

Today, with many races postponed because of COVID-19, you can still hear the positive words of encouragement that you listened to and have gratitude that you've finished the race. Carrying the good feelings after a race can be different for some runners, and if you feel fine after the stress on your body, you can start to run with intensity in three weeks. For example, if you read news in the newspaper and look at the pictures of the stories, it can help keep your perspective and attention on your running to help stay focused and not lose track of your goal.

Something that might motivate you is to grow in your field or career. If you are a business person working in a company, you can get promoted, such as a cashier at McDonald's or at Ralphs who gets promoted to an assistant manager or a financial analyst that gets promoted to a finance manager.

Hill training can also improve your average pace while racing if your goal is to get a certain qualifying time for a race. To qualify for the in-person Boston Marathon, you need a qualifying time in your age group; or to qualify for the Western States 100-mile run, there's a qualifying race to enter the lottery.

Today in California, there are many people who are ahead financially, emotionally, and physically, and it's a place where many enjoy life to the fullest because it's the sunshine state. I motivate myself by looking at some of the achievements that I have completed in school or in running such as with my MBA degree or my Series Runner medals, and the important thing to do is not to compare yourself to others. Once you stop comparing yourself, you can feel that the goals you set were achievable and that the mirror where you are now can accept the facts that running comes in many forms. Your focus on positive things lets you know your limits to know not to set yourself up in any way and know your fitness level is distinctive.

Some runners have found ways to continue to run and rehabilitate in their neighborhoods to keep physically and mentally healthy. Runners joining various races and running clubs in their community lets them participate together and log their results to see. Runners often make sleep a priority when preparing for races and is important to find similarities with other runners in how they prepare for a race to help you practice and plan. Also by knowing your own habits, you find ways to improve some bad habits. One of the important things that I learned is to set goals, hydrate, train, stay upbeat, and relax to run.

Today, the most successful politicians can interact with others by speaking at local universities or colleges to improve people's quality of life with their speeches and discussions. The runners who prepare themselves through proper training can be so healthy that they can blend in almost any environment. A runner can improve their image of themselves in public with more routines in the community to prepare mentally as well as physically well enough for their race. When I visit places while working, I feel a sense of togetherness with the people I meet that makes it a productive day, and while running, I try to find balance and peace on my course.

The many positive people walking, running, cycling, driving, working, and talking during a virtual course makes it clear to me that the world operates in an easy-to-read way if you go running. In your own journey, you are similar to the hundreds of other people that you come across with because you have a clear path to victory and can choose a route that is safer.

In a race that is in person that you register for, before the runner get to the starting line, he must enter the parking lot, which can get blocked off more as you try to find where to park because of the closures. I usually set my alarm and wake up in the morning, eat my breakfast, get all my items together to run, do an errand, drive to the race, go to the parking, go to the area where other runners are gearing up, and get ready for the run with a light jog and stretching to the starting line. Once I get to the starting line, I communicate well enough to meet other runners, which gives me lasting confidence during the race, and with the volunteers to finish line to get my medal and possibly eat before the drive home.

In virtual and real-world event running, there are beautiful surroundings to endure, and it often costs less to run virtually. Time with virtual running can be seen differently because the runner can start to run in a familiar area and motivate themselves to run well within the race's timeline. There are no volunteers in a virtual course and no aid stations, but there are people in the surroundings that can seem to help you as a volunteer or event staff would. Some of these people might actually root or cheer for you in your run and give words of encouragement for you to run faster. In a path on the beach, there are many ways walkers, lifeguards, and cyclists participate to walk together, and oftentimes the beach emergency vehicles and police cars patrol the walkway for safety.

Many of the Southern California races have beach themes, such as the Surf City, Long Beach, and Orange County marathons where runners can participate in challenges through the beaches. When I decide to run a virtual run through the beaches instead of traveling to the race, I still run through the sands—seeing volleyball players, surfers, bodyboarders, lifeguards in lifeguard stations, children with their parents, restaurants, fisherman—to experience the Beach Cities Challenge in a different way. The marketing and communication that goes on before a race to actual race day lets you feel safe to trust the marathon, and you often need to sign waivers before the race for risk of injury.

When running a virtual race, your time can be slower than the previous races; and it's often because when you run on a course designed for marathon and there are volunteers, there is added motivation to run faster with the other runners. You can wallow at the finish line without the stress of the starting line because you are running on your own time and terms. In the virtual runs, you can run on your own and picture yourself to be on the course. My journey of virtual runs has led me to believe that I'm in charge of how I experience the event and when I'm able to run and how I record it on my own time such as with my GPS.

In my journey of finding how to run regularly and moderately, I've found that it improves my mental health and cools me down to let go of anger and stress. By cooling down and lessening feelings of loneliness and isolation, I spend my time around runners that is often socially engaging and entertaining. In being able to deal with mental tension races, it help me center my thoughts to concentrate on the present time; and by knowing I'll relax after the race, it reduces stress levels.

In the expedition of seeing what makes people run, there are many who run to lose weight, better their health, compete in races, or try new things.

When a person goes out to eat at a fast-food restaurant, they can see a cashier or server on headphones assisting a customer with their order oftentimes in store or at a drive-through. While exercising in the gym, a similar instructor has headphones on and is teaching the class. When a runner tries to incorporate what they felt or experienced in a fast-food restaurant or gym, they have the confidence when listening to instructions for their race, that people assist others for you to have a pleasant time. I've known many ways to stay focused throughout a long race with the preparation given to me by my instructors, and I'm able to run feeling the physical, mental, and emotional benefits of the sport.

Running with a forward motion can give you a sense of purpose and social well-being. I can manage my time well at my job with Uber Eats because I'm able to accept orders from customers to pick their food up at restaurants and deliver it to them. With an open road in running ahead of you, the road is set out with many pedestrians' walk signals next to them, and you can have fun to give your body a workout. When a runner feels purpose to be in the right place at the right time, they can run faster and do what their body needs to do to grow stronger.

The pauses a runner takes to drink water to recover or use the restroom doesn't ruin your performance potential. Influential runners are often survivors because of losing an incredible amount of weight, as I lost one hundred pounds since 2007. Enthusiasts also set records in spite of obstacles, and they grasp their day as it unfolds and run at a faster pace for a long time. Runners use proper strategies, such as eating healthy and working safer; and when they see the prize money for the top three winners, it entices them to win it. Try to envision yourself running as people see you at work when you're busy, and you'll know you have what it takes to perform well, get the job done, and enjoy your run.

Many decide to stop more in running, which is fine if you need rest, but if you are constantly stopping, it could be a sign of issues with pacing, breathing, physical or mental issues, and whether you live your own way or your influence by others is your own choice.

Influential people often shape the news and our society, and it's a way runners can see to make goals for themselves. It is easy to read about the influential people in society, and it is important not to make comparisons and make goals for yourself to grow. Goals in running take time to shape, and once they are met, you can feel satisfied when you accomplish it. Currently, I look to all the nearby local races that are feasible for me, and I race most of them virtually. It is pleasant to see the races that have opened back to in-person events because you have the opportunity to run in person, on the course, with people again. For a long period of time, many races have not been able to operate due to caution around the pandemic. The goals for me are often competing various running events in a series to get a certain prize or a finisher medal combing the race.

A good way to start your running journey is to look into the mirror and feel comfortable about yourself. With this sense of self-esteem, you can carry yourself past many upcoming runs and marathons because a runner needs to have a sense of purpose and belonging in their society to feel that they can overcome challenges. When you are in a fast-food restaurant getting food for yourself, you can look at yourself as an accomplished runner; look at the menu; choose a menu item with balanced fats, proteins, and carbohydrates; and function and recover well. The choices you make in eating a healthy diet determine your energy level and ability to run longer and smarter.

One way to go about your running journey is to find your comfortable zone and accept that some people will say positive things and others may seem extreme to you, but as a runner, your individuality is strong. With feeling more relaxed and comfortable around people most of the time, either with your workday or with running, your energy can push you more. Many runners including myself are constantly trying to avoid injury, and there are highs and lows to find the right way to run effortless and with ease.

The typical way to look at your training plan can be similar to how you look at choosing cars. Usually, a buyer wants to make choices based on their driving experience, the car, the color, and the model; and once you see the car, you can envision yourself with the new car with a test drive. With choosing a race, people are cautious to choose an appropriate race within a reasonable distance, what their goal and motivation for the race. When I choose races on the Series Runner website, I have a motivation that the race will count toward mileage needed for the challenge, and if it's a race that I haven't run before I can get to my first step, I am choosing the best race for me. In a race, the size and location of the race are also considered because when I'm ready to run, other runners seem excited on my sense of know-how, which carries me well to the starting and finish line of a race.

In a typical race, you can acquire an appetite for certain food while running, and with a high-protein breakfast, you'll have your hunger under control. From M&M's to chips to cookies, many races give runners an assortment of food or fruits that can be enjoyed responsibly. The experienced runner knows how and when to eat their snacks and eat consistently so they don't overload themselves but instead use the food as fuel to race better. The body gets hungry, and after miles of running, listen to your body's needs with consuming calories and hydration to replenish.

I carry other items with me if needed such as a cell phone charger, my ID, water bottle, keys, tissues, and sunscreen. Just by knowing you are ready to rehydrate, you should continue to hydrate as much as you can and fill up your water bottle in stations for your body not to become dehydrated. Since I'm a combo runner, I know my body needs food after each mile, so I adapt to the refreshments given to me by the volunteers and bring anything else needed on my own.

The runners who perform better with caffeine can be satisfied with endorphins from just a little bit of GU. I don't enjoy having caffeine before or during runs because it doesn't make my body recognize my effort. Some runners that don't add caffeine to their runs often have a higher risk of heart disease. Naturally, bodybuilders perform better because they are calmer and don't take in caffeine, and in running, caffeine increases endurance and causes muscles to use fat as energy.

The aspect of running that is fun is that you are releasing endorphins in the brain for a runner high through activity or physical exercise. Since I know my body has endurance to run to a destination, I can use my confidence in the real world talking to someone. Whether you are a beginner or a pro runner, you'll be able to set your pace and destination to the open road and forget stress and have courage. For example, if you have a hard time at some point in your life, you can feel content by setting course in your run to move ahead and live life to the fullest.

A runner can build confidence by taking a look outside when it is hot. While the sun is out, feel the light and use it as tool to run and improve blood and oxygen flow in your body. I also take vitamins, and vitamin D is known to absorb better with the sunlight to maintain bone mass. After the long hard run, the runner can relax and see the sun set and experience continuous improvements to run with a sense of purpose. The journey can be long and one that has the runner can improve many aspects of their life, which started from jogging to running fast.

There are always better ways and places runners train for strength, and by sleeping, your body can recover well. For example, a runner can prepare for a race with careful driving to learn how they focus better so they don't feel tired. While actually running, you can also build strength by knowing your body has worked very hard on the course and you can then feed it healthily. Also, if a runner chooses to train just by walking, that can be enough activity for the day for them to jog and later run. A runner can uplift themselves by believing they are strong enough to finish a race after being tired so they won't give up when they have a small body ache or feel like letting pain overtake their run.

In the journey of running, it can be similar to self-discovery and making positive change and using energy to meet people. Many runners meet various people in their runs, and others prefer to run by themselves. They find ways to think of the time they have to run in their journey. With long distance running, you are in the way of building your body with a low intensity to meet many new people and see the world around you. In that sense, your running journey is a part of who you are and how you can meet people. You can feel as though your fellow runners in a race are on your own page and let yourself improve your self-esteem.

Performance in running depends on your body, clothing, environment, form, and genetics. Many times, the fastest runners have genes that give them endurance-related traits. In the real world, a person often creates their own reality with their daily choices and their work environment. I create my reality by working two jobs, participating in Toastmasters International, writing, running races, and taking care of my parents when needed. I respect people, and people often respect me. When I run a full marathon in the morning, I try to pace myself slower at the start, conserve my energy, and then run faster for negative splits later in the race.

In your journey of running, look first within yourself and later for the support and who cares about you. If you have family, friends, relatives, and coworkers, you have a support system. In addition, if you visit restaurants or customers at your job, you are building a network through training, persistence, and determination. Runners that are confident perform stronger, and when I run my races, I know I'm there to run. As you are running, picture yourself with the support of your family when you see the outside crowd and volunteers, and later you'll remember your race more when you see your family.

In running, there is a way to find and keep your pace, whether you aim for five minutes or nine minutes. Once you're at a comfortable pace, try to maintain it. I listened to trainers and coaches telling me they respect me, and I've chosen a pace on a treadmill and ran it often for twenty miles, which helped me keep a respectable pace during races. As I start a race with a faster pace with my fellow runners, I keep a good track of them for the first few miles, and later I can feel comfortable once the twentieth mile comes because I'm still running at a similar pace. By wanting to improve my pace, I'm able to see how my body kept up with the work I did to get there. Runners can find ways to overcome challenges by using their resources, whether it is at a gym, a workplace, online training, or other means they learn to do better than most people.

The main point is to feel good about yourself and enjoy your run instead of feeling you've overtrained and worked too hard. Listen and trust yourself, have fun, and think positive thoughts because you'll see others are with you to enjoy the experience. In working on yourself in your daily life, you'll find that while running, your motivation and pace will show to improve as you run through the event staff on the sidelines with a sense of satisfaction and pleasure. I've found a balance of activities and a diet to finish my races easier, as I reinforce my confidence and pleasure for a positive and safe race.

Running is a sport that is different for everybody to adapt to, and it often takes six weeks to train. Some people have trained much less and have a different style than you, and if you find a level of training where you don't feel obsessed, it can work for you while others train in different ways that seems to work for them. When you set out to train, you'll find a number of other people similar to you in physical strength, and it becomes second nature to plan and adjust your food intake and find a logical path from the start to finish of a race.

In the world, many people such as stock brokers, life insurance agents, and financial analysts try help customers with an economically sensible path of spending and saving money. In marathon running, there can be discounts to sign up for a race such as promotional codes to enter to save 10 percent while registering for events and also optional training programs that cost a little extra as a path chosen. Try to choose one that you feel will help you run that is economically and physically feasible for a race and that can give you a "runner's high." Often the runner's high is said to come after finishing a race, and other times it comes while running at a brief, deeply calming state of euphoria. The instructions given at every place you go in a race could be seen as encouragement to learn to be yourself and have fun.

When it comes to running longer distances such as marathons, you can get a feeling that you are on top of the world. Once you acknowledged the people around, you can try to prove to yourself that your training has paid off and you are on your way to a faster pace. This pleasure that you get from running far distances is one where you can feel individuality and rhythm to carry your steps in your run.

In running as in daily life, there are systems to how things are proven to work. Some fast-food places such as McDonald's can help with recovery and better performance in later runs, and they give professionalism and courtesy to enjoy your meal. When you are running, you can tell yourself where to go in a race or follow the signs and volunteers to finish and perform well. You have the guidance of volunteers who seem to know how to crack any code because they give you water as hydration and snacks to be there with you on your journey.

When a runner has a path on the road ahead of them, they can get ahead by figuring out the best pacing techniques to run throughout the race and to avoid cramps and exhaustion. When a runner gets new shoes for a running gear, they can set their shoes with zero miles on their shoe tracker and plan on new ones every four to six months or five hundred to seven hundred miles. Nike has many new models that can often be difficult to get because of the availability. However, the search for better shoes can be worth it. I've bought new Nike Air Zoom Alphafly NEXT% Flyknit shoes several times at a Nike factory store that had the air pockets pop within a few months often during races, and I exchanged them for new ones to find Nike Zoom Alphafly Next Nature to work best for me.

The runner is able to start at a new slate with new shoes that prevent injury and later excel to find a pace the body follows and maintains to achieve more in life. My running experience has also shown that new shoes are a way to help you run faster, avoid injury, and support your feet well as you run. The difference in trail running and road running is that your feet are more on dirt and rocks in trail running.

A feature that runners should utilize more on their running apps is to know how far they are in their training programs in relation to their marathon start date. I often wonder where my local gym really was because with all the miles I've run on treadmills show me the same place whereas an app such a RunGo can guide me to run a route and track my miles when others just run. My intention is often to run fast and hard to put the run behind me, but the experience I get differs because I see the course ahead of me as time for myself to overcome my challenge, going on to my next task of the day. I improved my self-esteem when I was away from the gym by telling myself that the things that I'm doing are healthy.

If it's your first time on a course, it can be a plan to learn and be familiar about it before actually running, through visuals at the expo or before the race; and if it's possible, talk to others about their experience to guide you. Most of the time, I'm successful without knowing the course as long as I communicate well and I'm as prepared as can be. The race instructions must be read before a race or at an expo because you can see some things that are different from your prior experience or the website itself.

Oftentimes the race director tells the runners they can survey the course before running or at least be familiar with where the starting line is before they run, such as what Linda Powell did for me at the 2021 Paiute Meadows Trail Run. The course map of a race helps you to find each mile safely, and it is often online or at the race expo or before starting the race. I view the course maps and try to have fun and talk with others to become familiar with where to go, and some races have their courses clearly marked and are easier to follow.

When a runner prepares to run, a long car drive to the race can be tiring. At my recent race, the 2022 Buzz Marathon, I took a look at the course map before the race and talked to fellow runners to see where to go. After the start, some runners made a wrong turn, and I also turned where they went, but it was only a few minutes of extra running. I also made a turn where half marathoners turned around instead of running straight, which added seven miles to my race and finish time. I felt the support of the race director Eileen Rojer, who said she was proud of me for finishing. The race staff gave me praise for finding the right way to go with resiliency and determination before finishing.

The level of your strength and the number of gains you make can give you time to plan to rest properly and have enough energy for your run later. Successful resting of the body is a continual effort and motion to recover for your body to absorb your training and adapt stress. In my recent 2022 Palm Desert Half Marathon, I was rested enough after taking two months off from physical races to finish a time just above two hours.

Running can bring people closer to you, which brought me to finish my first one hundred-mile Conquer Catalina Island Challenge, which consisted of running and walking one hundred miles on my own schedule and plan. In addition to running on my own, I pushed myself through my comfort zone to believe I was fast enough and had the time needed in the challenge to use walking at my job at Ralphs toward miles for the challenge. One hundred miles seems it would take a large amount of time and you'd be exhausted. However, by running and walking anywhere from two to six miles in day, I added my miles through the website throughout a few months to win the challenge. My running has led me to believe that I can train hard for a race, run well with my pace, avoid injury, and succeed in the journey.

I found the ability to see myself as a wonderful person and to respect myself and my overall appearance to show people I care. The running world has a lot of influential athletes, executives, inventors, and others who encourage us and allow our running lives. They deserve adequate respect to feel well. Running with a training program that keeps track of your shorter and longer runs can help you see how you've progressed with your training from the experience of the coaches in the training program. Runcoach gives world-class training for beginners and advanced athletes that lets me remember how I felt with each race because I write notes about my experience. The happiness that comes with the body naturally running stays with you for weeks or even month, and by completing running challenges, you are able to see your hard work pay off with more than one race. Medal races in the Series Runner Challenge are necessary to run to qualify for the medal at the end of the year, and as you log your miles with each race, you'll feel proud when finished after you earn your medal.

It is important to be happy with yourself to encourage others to improve as you excel toward self-reformation. I've noticed the whole world on my side, and by keeping myself on path, I listen to my body and make adjustments to run contentedly. The experience of getting a medal in a virtual race comes from running the race first, getting time to relax after you finish, logging your time on your apps, hydrating, eating, showering, and being in control when to submit your time. The joyful feeling stays with you from the photo you take of yourself to getting a medal in the mail. With virtual running, a runner can register and pay for a race, run the run, then take a selfie when finished. I send the results from my phone to the race submission link and, if needed, email the event organizer, and the event will send a medal.

In the runner's heart lies the secret to success, and there is a lot of feedback and stimuli a runner gets before, during, and after races. The better way for a runner to train is to have a start with a big picture view and have an end goal in mind, such as 26.2-mile race, and set a schedule that works and follow the plan from beginning to end. The gym can be a means for training well because you have a lot of equipment to use. However, runners can sustain success without the equipment that the gyms offer. For example, to train for an ultramarathon, a runner such as myself can run outside without a gym, but if a gym is accessible and you are in the facility, it can make your mental experience differ from being outside near the beach to see surfers in the ocean. By learning how to use a balanced running plan with a variety of runs and through meeting people, you can later rest calmly and with comfort.

In my journey of running and preparing for the start of the race, I often train somehow either at work by walking or with my running, and I expect to be comfortable on the race day. If I feel a cramp, I can easily get back on track in a race with walking a few minutes to later feel fine. A person with a strong ego can endure frustration, not feel selfish, and calmly solve conflicts, and every runner can find a stronger ego in themselves and respect each other. At one time, my feelings for the running world were neutral, and now I respect the fastest professional runners who are relaxed and have an honorable lifestyle.

A successful run can take time, and if you don't run too much, you can feel pain or cramps from the lack of training. Hill running can be harder, but success and strength come from keeping your motion at a high level. My body handles hills and cramping well, and my perseverance is strong. I try to run without pain by balancing my body movements and adequate training. A flexible training schedule comes in handy in situations that arise that make you need to run on a different day.

A runner can get back in the groove of running with smaller running goals such as running a few miles a day for a week before getting the groove back to run a marathon. When a runner wants to improve their pace for a run, there are several options that help. The first is having a workout routine that works for you so you don't over-train yourself. You could be running a marathon and see the fastest runners already on their way back and feel that you, too, are running well because of how you've trained. The next is finding the right type of diet to follow, and once you see results, such as a slimmer waist, you know you're eating right. In races, the feeling that I have is one of persistence because I know I'm capable of running a steady and fast pace at certain times.

The way I feel good about my running is through listening to the success I feel in my own mind after completing my runs. I'll tell myself during the run that I'm on my way to the finish line and that once I finish, I'll be proud of myself and I'm capable of rest and much more. My body feels different after each run, and it is important for you to feel comfortable. The joy of running comes from a runner's ability to see the running world not just for the run itself but also for its rewards. In my journey of running, my rewards are earning medals, ordering pictures, and feeling mentally and physically healthier.

The running journey can start with how you feel inside, and from there, you can build your moral to keep healthier. If you feel special enough to motivate yourself for a marathon, you are able to find ways to keep strong in your runs. Most runners that have not trained can often have a slow pace because they just want to go out for run, which can lead them to the hospital, but it can be a point where the runner wants to make more changes for themselves, such as to start walking or jogging. The way my training has work for me is to have a goal of a constant faster pace because I know I can run throughout the whole race. By looking forward while running and knowing how some people are slower, you can resist the urge to look back and focus on success.

Running can release hormones that boost energy, which is important to find if you feel tired because you can go for a short walk to keep energy. Running while you're tired is often something to avoid, and by saving your energy, you're able to perform better in your marathons. The way running has your body in motion is a pleasant feeling because as you run outdoors, you are communicating with nature in one way or another. Once you register for a race, you can add it to your calendars online to let yourself know how much time you have before your race to train properly.

Some calendars I use are Runcoach, Runkeeper, Future (24 Hour Fitness app), RaceRaves, and my Yahoo calendar, and I become a better friend and know how to plan better to travel for a race. The running events you sign up for have a lasting impression on your character because these finishing times can be achievements you can later see for yourself on the computer. In the Surf City Marathon, the theme is surfing; and since I mostly used a boogie board as a younger kid, enjoyed the waves, and sand, I'm familiar with the beach etiquette. While I run the race with hundreds of people being near the beach and seeing the sunrise, I feel accepted into the running world because of the theme of the run.

The part about running that can keep your mind open is to accept the race's name and theme as a means to put forth your effort and training for the end goal of seeing the finish line. The way to train for a marathon can vary from person to person based on their experience, as beginners focus on finishing the course and the more advanced runners try to finish in a certain time. I often try to run as many miles comfortably beforehand or with running groups to get a certain finish time.

Strength and conditioning can improve your chances of finishing a race with glory because your fitness level is strong. Race announcers often mention the experienced runners who have proven themselves by finishing in the top three or are sponsored beforehand to motivate some runners to make it through the race. For example, in the San Francisco Marathon, Jorge Maravilla won the race several times, and as I heard his name at the starting line of the marathon while running the ultramarathon, it gave me inspiration. I've also seen how fast he is in relation to my run because after a race, the race sends me my results and shows me where my friends are in relation to me on the course. Jorge was much faster than me and one of the fastest runners. Some runners choose to look at the sport of running as a hobby, which is excellent, and some find it to be more than a hobby, such as a best friend who feel special finding a light at the end of the tunnel and have a privilege for letting your body feel healthier.

The runners that make extra effort and plan for a race well will see that their training pays off with their finish time. With each race that I sign up for, I try to find a feasible plan to get my medal. In addition, I find ways that are financially easier from last year's effort, such as with my 2022 Series Runner Challenge. I'd rather drive to races in California instead of spending money for airfare when it's not necessary. In running a race, your body adapts to how you perceive yourself with the runners around you.

A well-balanced diet is one of the most important aspects a runner needs to follow to perform well. It can seem that while you are in excellent health, a burger with cheese or a slice of cake can bring your body out of optimum performance. Some of the fastest runners often indulge in burgers and fries after their runs as a way to celebrate, which is fine if it is occasional. In my diet, one thing that comes to mind is that what comes in your body later comes out, and a diet with unprocessed meats, fruits, and vegetables works fine for me.

When there is cake around in major life events such as birthdays, holidays, and wedding parties, it can often be a wise decision to just refuse it. However, when the body has sugar, it can often burn it if it is eaten occasionally, which makes it okay to indulge occasionally. The body has a way to burn calories with foods that contain fats and carbohydrates while running. The occasional feeling to eat what others often eat that make them overweight can be okay if you are consistent with your diet and exercise.

I felt accomplished to receive a medal for completing the Golden State Challenge Series, and it increased my pace from my normal runs. By having the consistent pace of about twelve minutes per mile in the local hills surrounding where I live, I've been able to have a certain level of confidence when it comes to running with a faster pace because I can conserve my energy throughout the race. The 2022 Golden State Challenge includes a combination of four races from a list of six to give you a special challenge medal at your fourth race that has a bear in the center of it.

In California, even the wealthiest individuals often need to leave the state because of the cost of living, but by having a medal that has bling can get you recognition for your effort to run in California. With series rules for 2022, the race has put virtual options for some runs, and it's enticing to complete the challenge each year when I can.

The feeling that comes with completing one of the most exclusive series of runs is one of proudness after getting through the challenge. In the Golden State Challenge race series, the Surf City 10 is one of the races that was completed by me virtually, and with the choice of running virtually, you don't have to travel too far and can run on your own time. In today's times, with COVID-19 shutting down businesses, restaurants, and many races, an individual can often feel overwhelmed because of the bills they still have to pay. And if they lose their job, there are more things that they must do to earn a living and survive. With running, the body is naturally releasing endorphins to let the runner experience bliss, and there is a once-in-a-lifetime opportunity for the runner to recapture their self-esteem and confidence.

With the other races that constitute the Golden State Challenge, the Surf City, Run Sip Santa Barbara, Run Sip Napa to Sonoma, Surf City 10, Long Beach, and Golden Gate marathons are other races that let the runner complete either virtually or physically. With a full marathon, or in my case a virtual marathon, the runner is able to have the opportunity to run their marathon on their own in an any setting or place. In life, many people are able to work for themselves to make a decent living, and many others have situations that make it harder for them to achieve what others have. There are barriers such as time, work, and disorganization that runners must overcome to be successful, and running enables me to break through most of these barriers.

There are ways that running or physical exercise is added for students in school to let them feel more well-rounded. In high school, there was PE or physical education that lets a student participate in anything from handball to running with a baton. Even in professionals' offices, there are breaks that employees get to use to feel more relaxed or to get any type of physical activity needed to achieve.

Another race in the Golden State Challenge that was completed by me was the Santa Barbara Wine Country Half Marathon. This race was going to be a two-hour drive for me if it was scheduled to be in person, but I chose the virtual option. The race let me experience a feeling of satisfaction for completing the run on my own instead of driving a long distance and purchasing a hotel room, and oftentimes the race gives the virtual option a few months before the race date.

As a part of the Golden State Challenge, the Surf City Marathon was an exciting experience since I recently ran it virtually, and because it is in Huntington Beach, and it's one of the more famous runs in California that lets most types of runners compete.

The mental illness chronic paranoid schizophrenia, which affects 1 percent of the population, has symptoms such as delusions and hallucinations, and in my running journey, I've learned to overcome it to be in partial remission through medication, psychotherapy, social services, and employment. With the first episode of the disease in partial remission, there have been tremendous improvements where I'm doing remarkably well, and there are no end points to be more normal. A person who is autistic can seem a little bit slower visually or even mentally impaired in social settings. However, with all of the advances in today's world of psychotherapy, neurology, psychiatry, and other types of therapy, most diseases can be kept under control.

In the media, the wealthiest people such as Elon Musk of Tesla appear to be happy, but they have challenges of managing their own health with diseases such as the coronavirus. They often maintain residence in California, but because of the cost of living or tax rate, they leave, which is hard to believe.

Series of running such as the Golden State Challenge lets runners overcome a challenge to see how the media and the wealthiest of people have had struggles with headlines of the news. To maintain positive exposure in the media, they need to continue successes in their business planning, but they leave the state or their girlfriends and let others see the opportunities.

A similar example of how running can help you overcome challenges is to see how it has helped some overweight people find ways to lose weight when all other areas they've tried have not worked. When running, you can sense your body often breathe heavy to keep you at a comfort level or pace. When a runner such as myself needs to get proper hotel arrangements for a race because it is too far of a commute, it makes a difference to get some extra sleep to perform with a better pace. Just as a CPA candidate is told they should have proper lodging before the test day to take the CPA exam to perform well on race day, a runner should carefully plan their race to get the sleep they need before the run.

In running a successful race, the atmosphere of a race such as the course and weather is important for the runner to be familiar with before the race to prepare and perform better. The runner is usually given a lot of applause and feedback by volunteers and fans cheering while running, and they are able to keep a faster pace if they save energy throughout the race. In virtual run, your finish time may be a bit slower than if you ran on the actual course. However, you can have a similar experience to the actual run if you can imagine your efforts to be on course.

With trying to find my motivation for running, it becomes evident that the structure in schools while growing up and throughout graduate school have shaped my discipline toward seeing running as an activity that creates more success with the hard work that it entails. At Silver Spur Elementary School, by remembering how to write proper sentences on paper and through the guidance from the instructors, I was on the right track because of my environment. I felt able to learn as many other classmates had even though I was born in a different country.

Throughout my junior high schools, one at Malaga Cove and one at Palos Verdes Intermediate School, I was able to stay active with intermural activities and with other students to see how the physical activity put me in the year book as "crazy legs." With this type of image and my own ambitions when high school came around, I tried out for the Peninsula basketball team to find that I didn't make it because others were so much more active and better at shooting hoops than I was. However, in college at El Camino, Los Angeles, Harbor College, University of Southern California (withdrew because of episode), and California State University Dominguez Hills, I still exercised with weights, played basketball with friends, and even played baseball.

In a dream class at a well-renowned school, California State University Dominguez Hills, I had the structure necessary to turn my life around by using my own intelligence to apply to schoolwork. Near the end of my school career, with learning, reading, and writing, my mind became more disciplined to eat a balanced diet and cut out the junk food.

Runners will often be told that they aren't doing well on a course, but you should take it as constructive criticism that you are because most of the time, if you keep running, you'll get past the words. I hear runners telling me things that I should lose some more weight to perform better, or other times, I look slim and athletic. With keeping a safe distance, I can hear compliments such as how good I'm doing. Many racers from the LaceUp Running Series have told me at the starting line of a half marathon to finish a race in under two hours. It seems easy at that time to be healthy at the starting line because of the way you trained. By seeing the fastest runners, you don't know how they trained, but you can be friendly and discuss running the race at a pace.

Train as you feel is right. Don't start off too fast or too slow, but listen to your body and guide it through the whole race. If you train at a gym, you can talk to a trainer and ask them how they've trained or see what advice they have to give you if it is within the budget. If you are in a situation where you feel that you have to work harder to get to where you want to be, just imagine how much you've trained to get to a healthier weight, and you can tackle the problem right away. Just as in running and with working, there are many instances that shape how you are able to feel later, and it's important to take steps back if you need to.

With being a combo clerk or cashier at Ralphs, it is interesting to see how the interactions with customers are ways to live a life that you dream of. If there are affluent people that you help with proper customer service, you can often hear things that can seem out of place or things that you can work on for yourself. Similar to how to properly motivate yourself in a run when you are at the starting line of a race, you can see many people are in three-hour corral times or faster.

When you are running a race and you are given a corral number or letter to start, that's chosen from your projected finish time from a previous race. In most of my races, I often go to the start of the corrals or the fastest corral to get a faster time. If my average time for the Long Beach Marathon was near four hours, I would step ahead to the fastest corral of two and a half hours to three hours to finish the race faster to start with the fastest but not usually finish with the fastest but maybe finish fifteen minutes ahead of a slower corral.

Successful and affluent people are white-collar workers and often live satisfying and happy lives with running, and I enjoy reading about those people because it gives me motivation. Marathon runners and people who exercise can earn more money than the average person. I've run more marathons and put in more work than the average gym member has because I knew how to run on the treadmill, exercise with weights, participate in classes, and find my way through my gym. Running races often helped me overcome the social pressures that arose at the gym. The course of a marathon and the gym atmosphere can be similar, but I focus resting after a marathon instead of more exercise to refuel and recover properly.

Oftentimes the experience of being in the fastest corrals is that most of the runners often can finish in the time for their corral. It is important to know your body's limits, how to adjust to the hills, and how to breathe properly in a race to keep a constant pace. The fastest runners run in race can feel proud of you to see you are running to the area they just came, and by having your body regulate itself and pause, you can feel that you are a successful runner.

In the motivation to run races, the body and mind can feel deep personal awareness and positive self-perception to heal better and faster when you train and recover the proper way. To train yourself properly, you need to carry your motivation and cut out your negative thinking. In the working world, there are customers that shape your day and managers that give guidance, and when you meet someone, you can improve your self-esteem and self-perception with your impressions of them by balancing your daily job. You can use your power of running and see how the successful runners make time to run daily and still have jobs that make them happy.

My end goal of running is to run and earn a faster PR or personal record for a course that I've already run or to be happier, healthier, and more successful. The goal of better health lets me work daily on eating a balanced diet, low in saturated fat and high in protein; and when I walk, exercise, work, or run, I know that my health is getting better. Also by finding more meaning with your goals such as what it means for you to complete a challenge, you can find that once it's complete, you achieve the medal yourself and not to meet others' expectations. Your body reacts to your effort, and building endurance while physically and mentally fit during long distance runs can give you inner peace and allow you to run with a constant pace to complete a challenge.

In long distance running, registering for the event early can save you money and time because most races increase their price as it comes closer to the event. Upon registering for an event, on the event website, there are options to purchase special jackets, coffee mugs, parking, and the option to engrave medals. A belt bucket could be earned for a very long run such as the Western States 100-Mile Endurance Run if you run in less than twenty-four hours. Free items, items on sale, additional medals, or a bottle of wine can be given after a race. A bottle of wine was given to me and the finishers after the 2022 Buzz Marathon in an army base room near the starting and finish line of the race in Camp Roberts. Runners often deserve more than a medal with their travel, and the added recognition from the race staff and others before and after the event is important for the community.

To run without injury, you can run smarter by taking a day off running every week or, even better, take two to three days off between each long run. The combination of running the actual run to later earning a medal are ways runners can maintain the feeling of accomplishment. In being able to maintain a pace through the start of a race and later throughout the race, a runner can find themselves to earn a very fast time. In my experience of maintaining a faster time, there are so many factors to remember before a race, and throughout the race that you feel very satisfied in the event if you missed a few things in preparation for your race.

Running ease your tensions, and proper preparation for your race can start by getting your items together before you leave your home. Your normal routine becomes easier than the marathon day because you see how marathons are structured for the runners' well-being and for you to endure a successful run by the organizers of the race. The runner starts at home, makes it to the actual course, and takes pictures at the starting line and, if needed, throughout the run and at the finish line to have their memories portrayed well. Experienced photographers such as MarathonFoto takes pictures and delivers endurance photos to runners, smiling proudly throughout their race, and at the end, they can keep their memories and give them a chance to order and view their photos.

Brave running can let you feel courage inside because you allow more fun, improve flexibility, speed, and stretching, and a fast pace can keep your energy from going away.

One of my preparation tools before a race is proper nutrition with eating a balanced breakfast such as egg whites, bread, honey, breakfast biscuits; and if it's a marathon, I'll usually skip milk. Oftentimes the next thing to do is to drive to the race and meet the runners on the course or to take a shuttle to the start of the race. It can be easy to forget simple things such as turning off your parking lights or forgetting to bring enough nutrition to the course. As a runner, you will see many people that have trained in a different manner, and if you feel that running a certain number of miles per week works well for you, you'll find confidence that can last you to the finish line.

A way to minimize injury in runs is to keep a stride or pace that lasts you throughout the race, and if you feel your foot cramping, try to pay attention to it and walk or stretch it off. In keeping your running form smooth, you can move your hands and legs together to find an adequate pace. When you run and you are able to maintain an eight-minute pace, such as with my experience in many recent marathons, you are in excellent shape. When your pace increases to twelve to fifteen minutes per mile and for some reason you lose access to the training tools that you once had, you can find yourself accomplishing more than ever because you are starting from another point.

By knowing your body and the points where you should slow down to avoid injury, you'll feel much safer. In my journey of knowing that my shin felt swollen during back-to-back virtual runs, I decided to research how to get the pain away naturally. By finding a way to avoid injury, I realized that by fast walking or slow jogging that blood can circulate better in your body and legs and you will heal naturally. My shin did heal without getting a doctor's orders, and by finding ways to avoid injury through reading, I healed myself.

In keeping safe and injury free, you shouldn't do too much too soon, but you need to train adequately enough to find comfort. Control comes when you're in a calmer state of mind, and others often sense that your time and actions toward your runs paid off well and happiness comes along with a new medal. It is important to be calm, workout, walk, and run to maintain a healthy mental attitude. Enthusiastic runners are committed to running, have goals, and enjoy their friendships when racing. The journey of running proudly and getting your medal comes with an extra sense of satisfaction that you know you did finish the run and you are entitled to good food and to have fun either by talking to runners, listening to the bands, or however you feel necessary.

In running, there are many ways you can become grounded if you look inside your training method and diet. Oftentimes you are calmer around others because of meditations and how you interpret the day ahead. In the running world, there are ways to live a healthy lifestyle even after your race, which comes as a second nature if you eat protein after your race. To maintain healthy eating and living, look at yourself mentally and physically stronger after the race because you are a kinder person through recognizing feedback. In running and later getting medals, the runner usually feels satisfaction as second nature because their bones get stronger as they observe their surroundings and familiar people.

I keep my medals hanging on hangers in my room, and I have four, soon to be five, hangers on my wall. I purchased additional bars for one hanger several times, and I've learned the best feeling is wearing your medal right after you finish your race. I usually take the time to wear the medal for fifteen minutes to an hour, and I hang it as a lasting achievement in my room. With all the energy of walking and running that goes into getting a medal, you need proper hydration before, during, and after the run to succeed. After you've gotten your medal, you can get back to your basic life and go home to rest or to work if you feel fine.

Training measures how long you spend running and how hard you train each week to see your effectiveness in your marathon finish time. It's easy to see that the more you train each week, the more energy you're burning and your marathon time will improve.

In the journey of surviving the cost of running, know that most of the time you don't have to pay because it's free. The important part of managing your money is to spend within the budget, and if you feel fine, you have made a wise choice or investment to become stronger and, in the end, get a medal. I pay for most of the races I run because I enjoy the experience of competing both virtually and physically. I can go out for a walk or run, but most of the races I register for are races toward a series challenge, which makes me live more. If someone is a fast-enough runner, sponsors can pay them for running and advertising, and they could win prize money for being the top three fastest, which is fun and exciting for other runners to try to get awards.

A runner puts forth marathon effort because they've trained a long or difficult task. After my training, I feel empowered to push myself harder in my training for an adequate, above average, and often successful race. In the long races, other runners and I push throughout the course to keep a constant pace while some exhaust themselves and are at the side getting medical assistance often from being dehydrated. My hindsight lets me keep my momentum because I know I've spent several days, weeks, or months to get to where I am to continue my efforts to get to the finish line.

Runners can find a better relation to the world to find that they are in touch with the environment the way they see themselves and how the world turns. As my running brings me medals, I see the time I spent trying to make things work better for myself in my daily and work life. As the age of a runner increases to forty, the time often slows very slightly on a course, but my expectations at forty-three don't slow me down because I work on oxygen uptake in my work-outs and stretching. A runner can believe they are capable and look very young at any age because of the health benefits added from their runs.

After long runs, a recovery aid, Epsom salt bath, can be used on your feet to lessen pain and help your muscle relax. By being an organized person and drinking a lot of water, a runner is able to get most of their work done well. A virtual run gives you the calmness to run when your mind wants to, and you know that if you were at the actual run in person, you'd run faster because of the crowd near you. The key to remember is to find a balance in diet and exercise that works for you. Don't exhaust yourself by the time you get to the starting line. What your body takes in, it takes out. Run with the present moment, and remember that you'll get to sleep later and resume to be more active the next day.

In virtual, I run the viewpoint that I run my course, and I know where I am and how far I need to go in the challenges that I participate in. If you've been successful in areas of your life and enjoying the moment when running a number of miles, you improve your outlook and frame of mind. The journey of feeling well inside or knowing yourself can relate to your running and how you've lost weight or got stronger when you know your body needed change. A recovery run can help twenty-four hours after running at a hard pace to give yourself time to rest. Usually after longer runs, your body can rest back to normal with an early run at sunrise or sunset, and nature is a place to go to feel better mental awareness.

The body's first mechanism to heal with recovery is resting in your run. This has shown me that my body gets a head start at situations on a course where I have time to rest at work, at a doctor's visit, with family, or with my recreational activities such as walking my dog or eating dinner. I feel that the more sleep, the better I'll feel the next day, and with a six-week recovery time from a surgery, the rest feels needed to repair my muscles. The joy of running comes with the sense that your body goes into a pilot mode before, during, and after your run to reduce stress and support your immune system. Oftentimes, symptoms of restlessness and drowsiness arise with watching too much television, not taking care of your body, and watching the news, and you need to find ways to stretch and drink more water.

Runners can sense the joy that is self-created by their choice of how they want to spend time training and choosing the various races they want to participate in. I chose many virtual races with little rest when racing, and now I choose to space out my runs form a series to enable a completely successful recovery. Many times, there are a number of races to choose from that often don't interest the runners because of time and money. The races continue to remind you of registration through email for you to either register again in the future, remind you of the event details, or congratulate you on being a part of the event because the prices increase. My preference in registering for races is to have either a series that is close to where I live, a series that offers a special challenge medal of nearby races, or a series that is accessible to run virtually and physically for a new medal.

The way runners have flexibility and freedom in races is pleasant, and it's important to reduce injury risk with rest and time for your body to repair, which motivates me to reach a new plateau in running or a new PR. By increasing my pace, earning a new medal in a new series, finding more comfort in the courses, and dealing with long-term injuries, I'm able to improve my mental and physical clarity and get rest longer when needed. I'm able to cross my next plateau in running through giving my brain a rest. Oftentimes it comes from stress relief while on the course and letting my mind relax, which makes it a goal to feel positive aspects of my character.

When I register for a race, I can decide to put more or less for training if I have a busy work week because many runners have careers that give them the opportunity to run before or after work. If someone does not have a job, that situation could be different. They could find some sort of balance with more running that helps with training. The media and coverage of running differs from the lifestyles that runners often live because most runners in the Olympics are shown as they compete, and when they are off camera, they live their own lives. The ability to feel strong on your rest days even if you are at work can help you if you decide to take two weeks off after a marathon to put your running shoes on and go for a run and compete with others again.

It seems to be true that runners in various marathons compete intensely and have a balanced plan of diet from the starting line throughout the middle and end of a race. The way training comes into effect is that if you are in a setting where most of your day you are on your feet, you need to find a way to make that time to train effectively with walks or runs. The activity of walking cross trains the joints and running muscles for a break to let you reduce aches and pains.

In actual runs, the runner is able to exert enough energy at the beginning to be able to get ahead, but later in the race, the runner can ease back a little because they are confident in their interactions and feel that they can run an adequate pace. The experience of running a virtual marathon brings about a reality in today's society that your effort will show to others as positive when you finish. The communication before, during, and after your runs will benefit you, and if you are at first questioning your run, later you will find answers.

In choosing a race to run, the runner needs to weigh their benefits first. In almost every race, the benefits are staying fit, less stress, working toward a goal, and feeling well with the community. There are many ways to enjoy your rest by taking time to recover and recharge your long-term well-being. In running and keeping high moral, try to portray your best self or mood, and later as you run, you'll pick up faster from your present moments by yourself. The benefits of running might not instantly appear, but you'll enjoy your time more on a run as you measure your progress.

Having better health, memory, and concentration through racing gives your mind a lift. The more you are able to adjust your schedule and learn and comprehend about how your body reacts during a race, the better. Usually after a race or within two to three months, I'll visit my primary doctor to get lab tests to pinpoint areas of focus with my body's complete blood count (CBC) to assess overall health and sense disorders. If a blood test shows one as being too high or low, I'll apply effective changes to improve performance through proper steps and feel much better afterward. Cardiac reactive protein (CRP) is a protein made by your liver, and it's sent to your bloodstream to reduce inflammation. Turmeric has natural ingredients to reduce inflammation, which is an immune response if the body or heart is inflamed from running too much.

It's wiser to take two to three days off between long-distance races for your body to reduce inflammation and pain or swelling of the affected area and not raise your CRP level too high. My CRP level was often high after races, and the inflammation went to my heart. I checked my levels frequently to find ways to reduce my elevated level, and I take at least two to three days off after a race to recover.

In running, as with most things, you can learn a lot and apply what you've learned later to live the benefits. There are several ways to be a better runner, and even if you are a novice starting to run, you can find ways to include a running schedule if it seems to benefit you. One is by being persistent with your running, and another is to improve communication while running. The running activity itself gives you as a runner time to feel energized and time to feel the mental activity that helps you recover well.

After a race, your body needs the time to relax and charge itself and improve capabilities as much as possible. The actual virtual marathons are exciting experiences because of the large variety of outside influences that help you attain your goals such as running clubs and series that are put together well. In my situation as a delivery driver, I can sense the times that I am greeted and understood well as a time to feel completely satisfied because I can connect with a network of people that are there for me.

While you are racing, you can sense your optimism on how people see you as talented and focus on opportunities instead of obstacles or what is wrong to use what you have and grow. If you are optimistic, you find what you're thankful for and use it at your desk or when you run in your community. The more you treat others with respect, the more you'll find others will treat you the same and will feel thankful for being at the event and for an exciting race. The self has a way of feeling hopeful by preparing for events, and by feeling healthy with a smile, you are on the right track. The runner that has a long and big smile feels calm and comfortable in their run and performs better if they hold it well.

The adventure of combining a healthy balance of food to balance your body for running after the phases of your training can show your body to get past certain plateaus. The confidence I gain from a run lasts a long time because it feels fine to just be in the moment with the music I hear and staying hydrated, which can be the key to a successful race from start to finish.

Running outside when it's cold can motivate you to be visible, and wear a beanie or jacket to keep the power to feel your potential and mental courage. I run most of the time when the sun is out, but it has rained and hailed when I didn't expect it, but it didn't discourage me because I protected my cell phone with my jacket and I had a fanny pack to keep my items dry. When it heats up, I feel a sense of well-being because I see nature and I believe in myself while running to outlast anything.

In a virtual course, there are many benefits of running hard to feel better for yourself. By running hard, one can achieve a healthy diet because mentally they are in more control to make better choices with what they eat. When running, the body gains heat after its active for an amount of time and can use it as fuel. The heat can help you get rid of colds and make your temperature normal or stable as you are able to maintain a better pace throughout your race.

In running, the mind and body work together for happiness. The way that the body endures the stresses of life go to the runner's advantage because your body has the ability to thrive well. In virtual running, the runner is able to picture themselves on a course as if they were at the real run, which can be special to experience in your community. The virtual race experience lasts long because in addition to your run, you also have time to submit your results online, get your medal and swag in the mail, and experience a pleasant event in a series.

My running improves with more mileage before a race, and during the race, I can keep a steady pace. After running, I feel special to have time to recover. The registration process differs for most races. Some require membership of a club, and others require waivers or prerequisites to agree with the terms and conditions before you pay. That motivates the runners the instant they register, throughout the run itself after getting your medal. It takes a lot of energy to start the run and communicate on your course, whether it be virtual or in person, and try to keep your conversation under control for better focus on maintaining your pace.

Your training can test your limits to finish a marathon if you took a personal challenge to run it. If you feel a sudden energy to run faster, you are on the right track; and if your body needs rest, take it in a proper way while still moving and running if you can. The body and mind work as you see people, and if you are tired, try running in place to lift you up. The hours I've put into the gym exercising, along with running, walking, and working, let me feel self-assured for the race and what it requires.

Viewpoints from others' perspectives must be looked at carefully to not let some social media websites lead to compare yourself with someone else's world because it can leave you with a baffled look to see if someone's careers and hobbies look better than yours. Some of the most successful runners spend most time running outside on trails, near their homes or in their homeland. The difference comes in your own level of self-esteem of how you feel as a runner and not to compare yourself to runners you feel better than.

I have enjoyed spending hours on a treadmill with running anywhere from one to twenty-two miles to meet my online training schedule that let me feel socially accepted and have a better outlook on life. Oftentimes from your training, you can get to run the actual race in four hours, and you feel confident that your goal is met because of the time you put into your race. By utilizing your resources of training to run a marathon well, you can look a little further to possibly finish closer to three hours from four. The fastest marathon runners and record holders use their own training methods of running near their country's origins, starting at a slower pace and finishing at a faster pace, running on coals or an allotted number of miles per week near their house to improve race times.

Runners can train simpler by eating better food, exercise, and running with a goal in mind of finishing a race. The experiences of getting to the race are often enjoyable, and by not getting anxious or nervous, you are able to keep yourself well prepared for a successful run on the race day. It might seem difficult to change to make the adjustment from driving to the race to actually experiencing others running with you, but running a consistent pace knowing you are going to finish the run is well-earned.

It is a big achievement for a runner to finish a marathon from start to finish line because it set you apart from the half marathon runners. When I communicate with runners before the race, I find that many of them trained weeks and some have barely trained, and I try to train at least twelve weeks. I feel personal growth and achievement when I'm mostly on the road. However, there are trails in many courses that certain trail running shoes are better. In some ultramarathons, the courses are mostly along trails and the distances can go up to two hundred miles; and gears, in addition to certain shoes, are poles that can help you in your running.

When you are on the computer registering for your event and later actually running the event, you can have a sense of satisfaction that you made the right choice and you'll feel excellent actually running. The courses and where to run in virtual runs are yours to choose from, by either running on the beach or running through the city. Being able to choose your level or intensity of running is fine, but getting a hold of your running style is essential for you to run well. The art of running can be a long-term tool to increase happiness and productivity as you use it to decrease stress.

The running sport requires you to stay nutritious to race when you need to. The choices that you make in life such as getting a driver's license to driving to buying a car can make you motivated, and while choosing running as a sport, you can go through the process to finish a race safely. The choices that the government gives young people are of importance because people want to live safely.

By feeling able to run, you are taking a step in your life to get up to where you want to be. A way to plan for runs is to get as much done as you need before the run and then have the mentality that things will improve and motivate you. I plan to run to enjoy the race rather than feel tired because as I save my energy toward at the end of the race, I can cross the finish line with my energy left. When a runner has a new found energy in running near the finish line, it's usually due to the positive environment, crowds, and the way the runner feels about themselves.

I ran and completed my first all-trail run called The 2021 Paiute Meadows 50K Ultra Trail Run, and satisfaction came after finishing the race because of the hills I ran. I researched ahead of time to make sure my miles would count toward the Series Runner Challenge, and I bought an airplane ticket, rented a car and hotel room, and felt prepared. One hurdle was to make it on time for my flight, and the security at the airport didn't let me in to my gate because I had a water in my bottle. They checked my bag twice and held it because I had water in my bottle flight, and I called my mom to find a way to get my bag through. I poured out the water, and they let me through. I sprinted toward my gate. I noticed the various other people at LAX waiting to get to their flight, and I just made it to my flight and asked the person at the gate to please let me in.

I still did not know if I would board the plane on time, and the employee didn't know either. After seeing the United Airlines hostess and saying my name to get in, I noticed that she was not running. I saw the standards of efficient work at the airlines to just let me make it on time. I picked up my rental car and paid extra for car insurance in case of liability in an accident. I drove to the race expo in Susanville, California, and I was given a special wooden model of the race in Susanville for my desk. The race director Linda Powell had to come meet me to set my app up for tracking on where I needed to go in my run.

After careful and successful planning on getting my running app to work, it made my whole experience in the race much easier because I knew where to go and didn't get lost. I kept a ten-minute pace for the first fifteen miles and talked casually with other runners about the success of being at that pace and on the right track. It was important for me to be on the right track to complete my run, make it back to my hotel to shower, and make it to my flight on time to return home to Los Angeles. The communication and timing with the runners and staff worked, and I felt successful to keep on the course.

The race had a hill called Heart Attack Hill, and for a moment, my pace went to eighteen minutes per mile, which I didn't expect, but I kept running. The hills were steep, and there were a lot of rocks. I had a faster momentum down the hills, and there were runners right behind me that told me I was doing well, but my foot and leg was numb or in pain.

Due to the generosity and kindness of my fellow runners, one offered me ibuprofen and his own water bottle to help ease my pain. My intent during the run was to just take the volunteers' beverages, which included water, ginger ale, Coke, and Sprite, and I know now I should have brought one extra water bottle. The run itself is a learning experience and allows me to continually run better and smarter. I asked the volunteers if I could fill my water bottle or if they could fill it for me, which kept me hydrated.

My pace increased to near seven minutes per mile because of my strong belief that my body shouldn't be in pain, and oftentimes you can acknowledge pain and not be affected. I saw a new movie called *Mortal Kombat* the day before the race, and I remembered how the superstars in the film were strong and how it related to my intent to run strong. By thinking of recent experiences with my family and occasionally letting myself go with positive experiences from my graduate school experience at California State University Dominguez Hills, I felt my pain was gone, and I finished with others and got a medal and was proud of myself.

The races that I travel to require light packing because I bring what's essential and I have an idea of what the race experience will be. I eat well, get adjusted to the time zones and temperature, and I try to sleep the next night well. I can successfully travel to other states for races, which shows minimal signs of a disability. Taking care of myself, I manage my finances well enough to come out ahead by the end of the year. The tremendous amount of work that goes into successfully running a long-distance event and later being able to relax or go back to work stronger can be worth your long efforts as you find ways to pace yourself. It is important to acknowledge having completed a marathon to recognize to not go back in time and to move on.

Runners communicate with you in many ways because they put in the same amount of work as you did. For example, my communication at the start, middle, and end of races is often about the time and commitment I've put toward the race. There isn't too much time to communicate with runners in the course as to the starting or finish line because you are spread out after each mile and I'm focused on getting through uncomfortable parts of the race in a relaxed manner. During the finish line area of a race, my style and confidence in words improve because I believe in myself and the goal doesn't scare me because I've achieved a feat that not too many have.

The unique aspect of many races is that there are alternate ways to post your time, and some races allow you to post your virtual run before getting your medal and swag. Some races allow you to run your race well before the race date and hold on to your time before submitting your results when the window is open. Some races require you to run your virtual race around a certain time frame because they accept race results in a certain time frame. The experience of getting your medal varies from race to race often because of the time frame to submit your results.

Running consistently on your own can improve your well-being through setting a feasible running schedule. I naturally find ways to figure things out smarter when I'm running on a course because my mind is free to accept and process the ideas that I've pondered. Many younger and older runners communicate with me while I work on a level for me to feel respected with my accomplishments, and I focus on setting new goals.

I've found many tools online such as social media, marathon training, and marathon websites to help me to show myself that I'm on the right track with my goals and training. In my recent physical run with the Series Runner Challenge, City of Laguna Hills Memorial 10K, it was a brilliant experience, worth the one-hour drive. Upon getting to the race and talking to Solutions table, I changed my virtual run entry to a physical run, and the communications were smooth before and after the race for me to have my physical bib held and picked up after the race.

I had pleasant interactions with the volunteers and runners before, during, and after the race. I had my own nutrition and picked up to a pace near seven minutes per mile by telling my body it had plenty of drive. By the end of the race, I remembered to tell the staff at the finish line that I was already given a medal because I ran virtually and I didn't order a T-shirt. I felt fine in the shuttle ride to my parking spot, and I updated my race apps with my finish time. I went to the 24 Hour Fitness gym after I cancelled my membership, and it made me feel positive to take care of myself and shower and enjoy my last month of membership before I no longer had access to the gym.

I worked with my former employer Postmates in Laguna Hills, and the restaurants and customers welcomed me. I got home to find about the nine races that I claimed results for from Athlinks, and it was a magnificent feeling to be up to date with my running and certificates.

In a virtual half marathon called the Round Valley Rambler, it was interesting to see that the race required me to wait until a certain time to run and submit my results. The guidelines were followed, and I found an open time from my jobs to run through the local beaches and complete my virtual run. I reviewed an opportunity to submit my results, and I did. I felt lucky to get another virtual race completed for Series Runner Challenge because I waited patiently to submit my results. The experience of the run and being able to look forward to receiving my medal is exciting because of having strength and taking the many steps needed to complete the race.

The way the sun rises and sets leaves me to catch the sun more so I'm not overheated or too cold. Overheating can come from a sudden shift in exercise style when you are breathing heavy and not hydrating enough. A way to reduce the heat of the sun is to use sunscreen, protect your eyes with sunglasses, and find a time that works well to run to beat the heat. Also when it's cold and your body adjusts to the coolness with more carbohydrates and drinks, you can try to bring an extra jacket to the start of the race that you can later throw away.

I've found a balance of happiness in running that comes when I give others a smile, a word of encouragement, or a high five. I keep positivity with the atmosphere in my race, and my goal is to keep life exciting because I'm not one person in a crowd. I find better habits of keeping healthy, such as eating less processed foods and red meats and replacing it with lean proteins such as fish, yogurt, or beans. I teach myself to be resilient and ask for help when I need to, and continuous self-improvements is a key to success that helps you in your community and to connect with others.

A smarter runner can see how well their body performs under different situations in a course. For example, in a marathon, there are so many aspects of the run that you need to pay attention to such as knowing where to turn and when to hydrate that you should have an idea of how much energy your body has from your previous training to finish. I found hydration by drinking a lot of water and electrolytes is the best thing for you in a race because you need more fluid to stay and run hydrated. My job at Uber Eats, previous job at Postmates, and my other job at Ralphs taught me to be aware and know how much water my body can handle at a time before I need to use the restroom.

Running without pressure from the outside world can be done with many steps to ensure your peace of mind. First, you must know who you are and what your goals are. Next, you must do things for yourself, at work, school, or at leisure, and take a look at what you need to later in the day. Setting attainable high goals in running can let you experience more in life and grow as a person and a runner. The physical exercise of running brings my body back to shape, and it's maintained because I'm able to communicate in a natural sense and vanish uneasy thoughts with the scenery and runners around me. By seeing various race courses and the efforts it takes to put on an event, it can bring an all-around sense of peacefulness when finish, and that can stay for a long time.

Bringing your belongings before your race should prepare to manage yourself physically, financially, and mentally before getting to the starting line. Shoes and clothes are vital if you're taking a trip because if you forget them, you'll need to buy them elsewhere. Also, when you have a flight such as the one I took from Los Angeles to Seattle, you should be prepared for the differences in people's attitudes because you are in an airport and your atmosphere changes as people try to make it to their flights on time. My passion with reading magazines and newspapers keeps me active and mentally sharp with my training plan when I hear feedback from coaches or others.

Some coaches say to run several miles a week such as a five-mile run a day or a longer run on a weekend. For example, a webinar I viewed with RUN365, which is a training program for the San Francisco Marathon, showed me that the coaches just want you to get your running shoes on and leave the house to run when you can, and if you can't make a forty-five-minute run, then at least go for thirty minutes. My training differs with virtual races because I have a set number of miles to run instead of a number of allotted miles that can be changed.

At the beginning of the 2021, by completing about three hundred miles of virtual runs ranging from one mile to 5Ks to 10Ks to half marathons and full marathons, I'm in somewhat of a different bracket of runners who train with twenty miles per week. I keep my excitement toward running because my runs are often longer than most training programs that assign a number of miles per week because of my virtual racing. I can run more races on a date that I can complete either virtually or physically instead of using the whole year in a training program to run one race, and oftentimes I keep active with a similar number of miles trained at the end of the year.

Registration for a race called The 2021 San Juan Island Marathon has been interesting because I received a special congratulations email from Active about choosing the race. I found out that I must get a ferry reservation from Anacortes to Friday Harbor, which I did through Washington State Ferries, and I needed to change my reservation because it would have been a gamble to try to drive to the ferry after my flight landed in Seattle, Washington, and make it to the race on time with the time my flight was scheduled. The next task for me was to get permission to go outside of my job at Ralphs after punching to use my computer and cell phone outside to change my reservation time to sail, and I did. I reserved another ferry to return after my race to make it to my flight on time, which I did.

The ferry sailed to the island, and I was mostly in my car watching the beautiful scenery of views of Anacortes to Friday Harbor island, getting ready to run. The San Juan Island Marathon was a pleasant and worthwhile race that I didn't believe was possible at one time because of the researching I did to find feasible way to complete the race. The race was my first out-of-state race, but it was filled with new opportunities for me to embark on such as meeting and talking to the race director Paul Hopkins to learn about the event and see if it would count for my 2021 Series Runner Challenge. After many emails and him talking to the CEO of Series Runner, I learned that the race would count, and I was motivated to run another in-person event, and I tried to space the in-person races throughout the end of the year to claim the highest challenge medal.

The first experience of my San Juan Island Marathon started when I drove to my hotel, the San Juan Island Hostel, after my flight landed, and I sailed in from my ferry. I got to my hotel and checked in without anyone at the front desk. I found an envelope and key left for my visit. I visited King's Market for food, which was the sponsor of the race, and I bought dinner and breakfast for the next morning and connected well with the workers at the deli and the market to enjoy the experience. I drove to the expo location at a place called Lakedale Resort.

It was where the bib numbers were supposed to be picked up during a certain time although the actual pickup times differed on the email to the runners and the website. I arrived to see that there was no one to hand me my bib unless I stayed at the resort. I met some runners who were in my situation who made light of it, and I enjoyed the moments because of making it so far. I was advised to come the next morning.

The next thing I needed to do for the race was to sleep, and I slept well. Oftentimes upon traveling for a marathon, I have a unique sleep pattern because I rest calmly and dream vividly with a pleasant reality around me and others because of my goals.

The next morning, I was ready to go to the race expo again, but first, there was a place called Friday Harbor High School where I read that I was supposed to park and find a shuttle. I arrived at the school, and there was one runner that was there waiting for a shuttle, but the shuttle was not there. I drove myself as I told myself I wanted to just pick up my bib on time. I was able to pick up my bib, and I saw an opportunity to go back to Friday Harbor High School to park my car and get the next shuttle back to the resort, and I made it to the resort to start the race.

I arrived to the Lakedale Resort with other runners with me on a bus and met the race director and many others outside. The staff was nice to meet, and they offered me words of encouragement that they'd see me at the finish line after the race. I viewed the course map, and we took another shuttle to the starting line. The starting line was by the ocean, and there were many questions that I had answered such as the types of hydrations and the way the course had four locations with restrooms. The race started after we took a group picture, and I made sure I smiled.

I met people and started running, and I ran with the three fastest runners after about one mile. My pace slowed to about nine minutes from eight and then to ten, then eleven, then twelve. I brought water with me this time and an ibuprofen in case I would be in pain, and I used a little bit of ibuprofen in the run as I kept communications with my Uber Eats employer through reading the text messages to see why I wasn't able to go online in another state or to see if a document I submitted has been approved. The pain was a little bit on top of my right foot, and I've felt it in other races and even in indoor cycling when I worked out at the gym. It was a sign for me to walk slowly to figure out how to navigate past the pain, and I did, and the pain went away. The other runners kept running and told me I was doing well, and the spectators driving thanked me for coming out to the race.

By leaving my cell phone on during the race, I kept my apps going with RunGo, Runkeeper, Runcoach, Nike, and my Future app. These apps kept track of my miles and pace running through the island's gorgeous seashores, nature trails, and wildlife. I remembered the shuttle driver telling me and the passengers before we got dropped off to the starting line that there was an airport on Friday Harbor that flies to and from Canada, but as of now, there is no service due to the pandemic. An agent on the telephone told me the same thing when I booked my trip.

As I ran, I was welcomed to Canada through a text message from Sprint, and when I called the number, I listened to the recording with bad reception, but I felt well to see that I was in another country after checking my text messages after my run.

Usually, to go to another country now with the COVID-19 pandemic, a person must quarantine for three days after being tested negative for the virus to travel. The race in San Juan Island was filled with friendly volunteers that assisted me with various nutritious snacks, such as bananas, M&M's, gummy bears, pretzels, Gatorade, water, and salt. I filled my water bottle with water and Gatorade to stay hydrated at the aid stations, and there were markers on the course that showed me where to go. For example, the volunteers showed me and the runners different pages with colors to view before the race. The color of the arrows were supposed to be green, and in the course, the color was closer to yellow. I made a turn that made me lose about ten minutes trying to find the right way, and I did with the help of a runner behind me telling me the right way to go.

The finish of the race was satisfying because I found my way at a constant pace. A successful race lets me feel my body, mind, hand, and feet movements are steady and fluid. Other times, one part of my body is a little bit slower or in pain or cramping, and I need to focus on keeping myself running throughout the pain by walking to get back to a comfortable pace. After finding an appropriate pace, I reward myself with a snack from the volunteers or drink water, and I feel the nutrition helps recover faster.

After the finish line at the San Juan Marathon, I was handed a pretty medal that I was proud of. I talked with fellow runners about their experience on the course and how they did, and they told me they ran well. The food choices of chicken burritos, chips, cookies, bagels, and peanut butter were delicious to eat after the finish line. There were shuttles that were supposed to take me back to my car at Friday Harbor High School, but they leave without me because I missed them. The staff told me it could be anywhere between twenty minutes to two hours before I got back to my hotel and car. I ended up talking to a staff member and arranged a taxi ride, and I felt grateful to make it back to my hotel to take a shower and leave to my ferry.

A successful day with running can take time, and if you take a four-week break from running, you can feel your muscles recovering well. To feel safe when running, try to keep your momentum and determination at a high level, and you can have more success when you get to the harder hills. In a marathon, you need to listen to your body when you feel pain or cramps, but your body can handle hills and cramping well. In my perseverance, I learned to walk successfully without pain by balancing my body movements. Being flexible to your training schedule when situations arise can help you make changes when needed. Running these events, choosing your own pace, and feedback from volunteers can improve your pace. My focus is on my mileage, daily activity, and to maintain a schedule for more improvements.

While registering for a race, there are often many distances to choose from, and it's smart to not choose a length that you can't run. If a runner has a course ahead of them, they can listen to music, and it can block out pain signs to the brain and reduce exhaustion. Music can also help you at work or in your car too and can be an extra luxury in your day. For example, at Ralphs, music is played. The customer can listener when they want and be familiar with the songs.

The body and mind react to other people while listening to music, and when you run, you'll feel less pain and just run instead. While I'm working in a grocery store, I can hear music playing while at other times, I ponder whether the music is there or not because I'm productive interacting with someone else.

I've run marathons with my Fitbit Ionic Flyers headphones, but I stopped wearing them because Fitbit discontinued them, and they had a recall on the Ionic watched too. I felt a sense of camaraderie with other runners because I had three different types of music to listen from Apple Music, Pandora, and Deezer, which all had running songs that I became familiar with. I purchased the newest smartwatch Fitbit Sense, which is an innovative smartwatch with many features that controls your health. When running with the Sense, I became familiar with the features, and I no longer needed to carry a charger with me while running, and I don't use headphones.

I prepared for 2021 Deseret News Marathon by slowly packing before my flight, and I requested the days off needed from my job at Ralphs. I let the management at Ralphs know ahead of time that I will be traveling. My job at Uber Eats is self-employed, and I didn't need to request days off or let the company know I'm traveling. The interactions before, during, and after the run were filled with many wonderful memories, and I was prepared at the airports with my ticket on my phone and properly weighed carry one bags. I arrived on time to Los Angeles International Airport and boarded my plane with my group letter, and I had the time to use my computer on board.

To prepare for the marathon, I tried to train with a long run three weeks before the race, and my virtual runs and mileage reduced before the race. I got more sleep for my body to be ready. It took time and preparation to get to the airlines, hotels, and to the starting line of the race, and I cast my doubts and focused on overcoming the challenges and to have fun. It was convenient that the expo was at the Marriott Hotel at the campus of the University of Utah, and my plane landed at the Salt Lake City Airport. I got an Uber ride to my hotel. I checked my Uber Eats delivery driver app, and since I was in another state, I needed to wait until I got back home to go online and deliver.

I tried to call a taxi at the front desk of my hotel to get a ride to the starting line at Rice-Eccles Stadium in Utah, and there was a chance of getting a ride, and I even changed my wake-up time to thirty minutes early in case there was no ride. Upon checking with the front desk at my hotel and looking outside, I saw no taxi was waiting for me. The taxi company said they had no drivers and there were no Uber drivers either. I chose to run and walk to the sports stadium and shuttle area to get to the starting line ten minutes before the shuttles.

I went through the university's campus at night, and it reminded me of collegiate life and how students participate in their school athletics to further their academic career successfully. I studied for my own graduate degree and earned good grades and worked with my professors after hours to ensure a successful class experience and an edge I can use in running and other part of my life.

I met some runners by the busses that were from the San Francisco Bay. They seem interested when I explained I traveled from Rancho Palos Verdes, California, to run in a marathon that would count toward the 2021 Series Runner Challenge, with an opportunity to run a combination of five hundred physical and virtual miles.

The bus ride was fine and dark. Upon the ride up the Emigration Canyon mountain, I charged my cell phone to a full charge, and I met runners and race staff at the tents at the top of the mountain. I felt inspired to discuss my recent achievement at the San Juan Island Marathon where I took a plane and ferry to make it to the marathon. The volunteers told me about the porta potties and that I shouldn't have problems finding restrooms.

Before starting the race, at the start of the race, I met a runner that told me that I should expect the hills to be a little harder on my legs. I stretched and used the porta potties, started the race, and the course started from the top of a hill called Big Mountain and went downhill for five miles, and then it had some hills to run upward. The hills were a little harder on my legs, and often I felt a little pain on the top of my foot, but I managed the pain to not have to walk. I took an ibuprofen, and the pain was under control. I ran with a pace of seven minutes per mile to later go to fourteen minutes per mile, and their police and volunteers on the course were directing the runners where to go.

Talking with runners before a race can give you a mental clarity and a mental edge that helps you find a constant faster pace. Keeping your mind in the present can keep your momentum to communicate with the volunteers, personal, and runners. A volunteer is performing a service of helping you with water or refreshments, and a service can come from two different sides or parties. Many people work at different levels at their lives; try to find an understanding. The volunteers at water stops and police officers guiding traffic provide a service and work for you and the race to run faster, and it can help you in future races.

I finished the race satisfied to achieve a time of five hours and one minute, and the race announcer said that I'm a machine who ran well. A medal was given to me from the volunteers, and I was congratulated. I felt it was okay to grab a cookie, water, a banana, and a sandwich without sauce from a Chick-fil-A bus nearby. The finish line area was set up very professionally, and there were many younger students in bands and younger kids who were cheerful watching a parade of floats that made my experience and weekend in Utah satisfactory.

I tried to get an Uber back to my hotel after the race, but I canceled it because I found a free shuttle that took runners back to my hotel and stadium, and I made it to my hotel room in time to shower and take care of myself.

I got an Uber ride from the Marriott to Salt Lake City International Airport, and the car ride was pleasant and filled with joy where I explained my purpose for my trip and run and learned about the Pioneer weekend coming up in Salt Lake City that represented their heritage.

In the airport, I communicated with the personal and gathered my items and scanned my E-ticket in the area I needed to when checking myself in for my flight. I updated my various running websites such as RunSignUp and Athlinks, and I found more race results to claim and downloaded more finisher certificates to print. I also registered for another virtual half marathon that was in the Series Runner Challenge because the series often has races added for runners to choose from.

While running a local Rolling Hills Estates 10K, I felt organized and self-motivated to get to the starting line, run by the nearby houses, see horses, and later at the finish. The next day I ran a virtual half marathon in the Series Runner Challenge called Big Brothers Big Sisters of Flagstaff Dave McKay Memorial Virtual Half Marathon. I ran by the local beaches with a pace of eleven minutes per mile, which kept me with a busy running regimen. I felt fine after the race, and the next day, I ran another Series Runner virtual event called the Fort Collins Human Race Virtual Half Marathon, and my body was a little slower perhaps because of something I ate a few days earlier. I went to submit my results, and I found that the event director locked the section for me to input my results. I sent a few emails, resolved the issue, and submitted my results. I worked with Uber Eats, and my stomach pain healed naturally.

Running can let you practice social skills, travel places, and let you write about your experience, and I often write a review on a website called RaceRaves where I describe the most unique aspect of the race. Improved self-confidence can keep you from getting distracted. For example, I submitted two race results in one day from the virtual race platform; one was Big Brothers Big Sisters Dave McKay Memorial Virtual Half Marathon through RunSignUp, and the other was the Dave McKay Virtual Half Marathon.

I wrote my review for the Dave McKay Virtual Half Marathon on RaceRaves, and I also submitted a review for my recent Hot Trot Virtual Half Marathon, which was run months ago and is a part of the AMPT Triple Threat Challenge. The window recently opened for the actual race, and my virtual run was months ago. I used my results in the window, and they were accepted. The AMPT challenge was also originally with Series Runner, and now the races are not still with the challenge. The Series Runner Challenge didn't accept my AMPT results because I didn't add the race on my Favorites in time. However, a medal including a shirt were sent to me. Also there is more incentive for a challenge medal to arrive after three races in the series have been completed, which is called the AMPT Triple Threat Series. I earned the new AMPT champion medal, and it was my surprise that the design changed. I was happy to get the new medal and felt like a champ because of all the hard work it took me to properly register for three half marathons.

I received some hard-earned medals in the mail recently, such as the 2021 California Time Travel medal and a Human Race Half Marathon medal, and my collection grew and I got more certificates to believe more in my overall health. I asked my primary care physician about the sharp pain in my foot, and he referred me to see a foot specialist. It made me feel fine to know that my foot appeared to be completely healthy for my upcoming 2021 Santa Rosa Marathon. I talked to my primary care doctor's office to find that it could have been a sprain, and I got ointment and over-the-counter medication to deal with the pain. Day by day, I felt better and better for my pain to go away.

As a spontaneous runner, I found that there will always be something that can steer me off such as gaining a few pounds or having diarrhea or a different kind of pain somewhere in my body. Glycogen is how your body stores carbohydrates in your muscles for more energy running on hills. When it has a high level of glycogen, fat, and carbs, it gives you a higher heart rate and you need to use your energy when running on hills. And when your heart rate is lower and using fat, proper breathing can help the body run with glycogen.

I was excited to get up early in the morning for the Santa Rosa Marathon, and I felt prepared for the race. My mom gave me a ride to Los Angeles International Airport and told me suggestions about things I could do, such as meeting other runners traveling through Santa Rosa. I arrived at LAX, walked through the gates, and showed my boarding pass to security without any issues. I landed in Santa Rosa and rented a car and traveled the city to see beautiful gardens, a movie, grocery stores, and ate healthy food. I was well hydrated, and I forgot to bring my running shorts from home, and I bought a new pair at the local Big 5.

I visited the Charles M. Schulz Museum and enjoyed the staff and artwork and watched the film of the late artist. The expo of the race was at the Sport Basement, and there was a lot of helpful volunteers. I was guided to pick up my items even though I already had my packet mailed.

I was offered wine at the expo, but since I flew there, I didn't take it because there would be an additional charge to check it on my flight back home. The marathon in Santa Rosa started at 6:30 a.m., and I met many people before the start, and I told them about my recent marathons, trail runs, and my expected time to finish my race.

I started at corral A, and I felt fine about starting on time with the other runners. I got my running apps ready to track my time. The course was mostly flat and went through many vineyards, which was a first for me in a marathon course. In addition to the vineyards, there were many cows and goats that were on the course along with beautiful trees and scenery. I communicated with the volunteers through drinking water at the stops and filled up my water bottle when I could.

When a gain is achieved in the stock market and earnings are made, the investor can decide whether to take out the money or invest it again. A runner can start running and improve their pace by taking steps inside the house, add a smaller- or longer-distance run outside their house, and then find it sensible to step further and register to run a marathon.

On the course in my recent marathon in Santa Rosa, someone asked me if I was playing the stock market as my training app for RUN365 finished the goal of about eighteen. I chuckled and kept running, hearing new opinions. There were various porta potties throughout the race, and some were lifted by a truck. I learned the way wine was made in a vineyard. It was exciting even though I don't drink alcohol.

My foot felt no pain in my race, and I was glad that it didn't because I kept a pace of eleven minutes and thirty seconds per mile, and at the end of the race, my name and age was called by the announcer. I felt proud to get my medal from the volunteers and to get some things to snack and drink such as bananas, Dole fruit cups, chocolate milk, and a granola bar. My experience in Santa Rosa City was pleasant because I shopped at grocery stores, ate a healthy lunch and dinner, saw tourist attractions such as the Charles

M. Schulz Museum, visited malls, visited historical gardens, participated in Toastmasters Zoom sessions, and safely drove my rental car. I updated my race results on my computer and started preparing my next physical race, the 2021 San Francisco Ultramarathon for my Series Runner Challenge, as I waited to get on board for my plane. I felt that I recovered well in lower back and hip pain from my Santa Rosa Marathon.

Running can have lasting effects on my moral when I start to feel like I can communicate with others without boundaries and a sense of self-gratitude and confidence with endurance events. I had my 2021 Headwaters of the Frio Virtual Marathon rescheduled to 2022, where $250 is needed to be raised for a good cause to helps a children's fund that provides food, clothing, housing, and transportation to restore the lives of abused children in need. After sending a donation request to one of my Toastmaster friends, I also got a $50 donation and $50 from my mom and $20 from my mom's friends. Running events in a challenge requires focusing more, thinking positive, and being natural and sensible while running. It can let you meet various people on the courses.

With virtual running, I need to feel athletic. After a negative COVID-19 test, I realized that I feel healthy, and I had fun in my 2021 Virtual PeaceHealth Appletree Marathon. I went out the door after asking my doctor's approval to run my upcoming San Francisco Ultramarathon, and he said no at first. I explained that I had no foot pain, and he changed his mind, and I was on target for the race. I submitted my results for the virtual marathon in a calm manner, and I felt energized and happy that I set my own pace.

I planned for unexpected events before making a trip to San Francisco for my 2021 San Francisco Ultramarathon, and the outcome was positive. The night before the ultramarathon, the race director sent out a welcome packet with guidelines to the runners in preparation for the race. I was working at Ralphs days before the race with early morning shifts and Uber Eats later in the day, and I maintained my motivation with people around me with feelings of deep personal awareness and positive self-perception. I bought the newest Apple iPhone from a T-Mobile store and ate dinner at Kalaveras restaurant in Redondo Beach with my parents. When I got home, I let my dog out, and she was bit by a coyote. I had to wake up early the next morning to board my flight, and my mom drove me to LAX, and I went to the terminal on time.

It is natural to worry about running a race without injury, and changing your feelings from nervousness to being full of energy can be done by shifting your focus to your pace. The run ahead can be very fulfilling and safe if you keep running at a constant pace to be satisfied because later you can take a rest, see a movie, go sightseeing, eat out, write, and read.

The journey of running can seem tiring, but you can plan on taking longer rests or breaks when you feel tired and sleep properly. I read different tips and methods to gain or sustain drive and confidence online, and I learn to keep invigorated when I run. Nighttime running is often the safest if you have a headlamp or a reflective vest, and usually you are one of the few people who are making that effort at night, and it's ideal for people who feel tired after running.

I landed at San Francisco International Airport and rented a car to get to the Sports Basement expo for the marathon, and it was filled with excitement because I met people that inspired me with their stories. I bought a small water bottle for my runs that fit on my hand that helped me stay hydrated and race without carrying too much in my hands. I needed rest before the race at my hotel that was reserved. I went to the official ultramarathon expo location or hotel called the Hyatt near the Embarcadero, and I checked in with the race staff and chatted with the runners about everything such as restroom locations and what to expect on the course.

I started the race at 11:00 p.m. and ran the first lap with my headlamp, and it lost its batteries at thirteenth mile, and my cell phone automatically called all of my emergency contacts by accident and was locked for about twenty minutes.

My time for my first lap was five hours and twelve minutes, and I had an hour and a half rest before the second lap. I started the second lap and received a lot of compliments from runners about being an ultramarathoner. The support of other fellow ultramarathoners was felt on the course. We kept together for about six miles to run stronger and pace together. I finished the race with qualifying time and became an official finisher because my time was six hours and nine minutes, which was lower than the six hours and thirty minutes cut off time. At the end of the race, I walked with other runners to meet the race director Michael Li at a nearby tent to give me my ultramarathon medal, and we took pictures and had fun.

I went to the Hyatt to get my items and drove to my hotel to shower, and on my way to the airport, I stopped to get healthy food at a Mexican restaurant. I caught my flight on time and flew to Los Angeles, and my mom picked me up at the LAX airport. I felt a new feeling of success and joy for my accomplishment.

In a virtual race called Girlfriends Run Virtual Half Marathon, I had to run two extra miles from my 13.1 allotted miles to log my apps on my phone, and I had the determination to finish due to bad reception at the time. In my morning, I participated minimally in a Toastmasters meeting while running, and since it was an all-girls race, there were no age division awards given.

My next race was run in person, the 2021 Denver Colfax Marathon, and it's Denver's biggest marathon. The race was rescheduled, and my mom drove me to LAX. Our conversation was toward family. The race is a Boston qualifier that goes through Empower Field at Mile High twice, through fire stations, and ranked in *Runner's World*.

My flight to Denver was with Delta Air Lines, and it was my first experience in a flight as a Delta SkyMiles card holder. It was a learning experience similar to other flights because I had to pay attention to safety features on board and get prepared to pick up my rental car, go the race expo, and go to my hotel.

In Denver, I picked up my rental car and paid less through my Delta card. I caught a shuttle to the car rental area and drove my car to the expo at the mile high Denver Broncos' stadium. In the stadium, I felt my back ache and feel weaker, and I got a massage with a massage gun and another by hand, free of charge. In waiting for the massage, I viewed an executive suite that is used to watch the Denver Broncos football team play, and they had a game the next day. I saw myself as a pro football player, and I took pictures and focused on the tasks needed to relive my back pain and finish the marathon.

I went to the race expo upstairs, and there was no reentry. I picked up my bib number and communicated with the race expo volunteers about the race day information such as parking and the Series Runner Challenge. They directed me to another information booth, and I talked to two volunteers of the race about my Series Runner Challenge questions, if they had a virtual option or if they were in the challenge or not, and they didn't know. I had the same chat about the Series Runner with the Denver Colfax race staff before signing up for the race, and they confirmed that the race would count toward my challenge. A staff member or a race director from another race felt that if the race has a virtual option, then my physical miles would not count. I explained that even a medal race such as my upcoming 2021 Seattle Amica Insurance Marathon must count toward the physical miles needed for the challenge, and he agreed.

I went to my hotel and found an Olive Garden restaurant to eat at for lunch, and during the wait, I picked up some groceries for food from Target. I felt some back pain that might have come from my front-end ripper duties while working as a combo clerk job at Ralphs because the management scheduled me for my combo clerk shifts. I was asked to come to work an hour early as a front-end ripper to recycle cardboard boxes, which was a lot of weight and could trigger back pain.

I gracefully picked up my lunch from the Olive Garden and drove to my hotel and emailed the CEO of Series Runner to ask him my questions about the challenge, and I'm fairly comfortable with my knowledge of the running series and felt successful in the challenge so far.

It was my brother-in-law's birthday, and I wished him a happy birthday. He told me to be safe, and I got seven to eight hours of well-needed rest and checked my work schedule at Ralphs and had no days off. I have an opportunity to earn adequate income with my other job at Uber Eats, but I'm able to handle any work changes and live a healthy lifestyle.

My alarm clock woke me up in the morning, and I brought basically everything I needed to the race in my fanny pack except for the sunscreen. I met other runners at the starting line, and it was very cold in the morning. I wore my Santa Rosa Marathon jacket to keep me warm, and if I feel warm enough not to bring a jacket, I won't bring and wear less from the start through the finish. I started running, and at the ninth mile, the lead half marathoner came behind me with a police car and bike and officials. I noticed he ran and picked up his feet high behind him with forward hand movements, and I've trained at my local gym feeling at his level and style when I was a member.

The various police and cadets guide traffic and help you stay focused to run faster. Keep your running goals in mind along with your body movements to continue find motivation to race safely. At the finish line, I ran faster because I had the energy and met many people who congratulated me. There were half marathon volunteers who had medals, and I was guided to someone who gave me my marathon medal, which had a beautiful design and words engraved that said, "Thank you for helping the race go on." I walked the wrong way to my car, and I ran to find my car with the help of others, but there was a miscommunication between me and the Michelob beer volunteers and race staff to find my car.

I experienced friendship with other runners who ran the marathon relay because they told me they wanted a better time, and I told them of my time and about the frequent hills but that the race was mostly flat. I also met a finisher wearing a Boston Marathon shirt that had a time of three hours and thirteen minutes, and he told me I did a good job with my run. I found my car and drove to my hotel, avoiding needing to pay an extra $25 for parking. I felt fine to just take a shower and leave, and I handed my room keys to the staff and also drove to fill my car up with gas before driving to the airport shuttle drop-off area.

I got a shuttle to the airport and called my mom to remind her of my pickup time at LAX with no changes. My mom congratulated me after my run, and it felt suitable to tell her my story of just eating two protein bars and stingers and that I had fairly normal bowel movements. I ate a healthy meal of honey mustard chicken sandwich from Quiznos at the Denver International Airport, and I updated a lot of my running apps with my results and showed my coach from Future my progress. She said my splits looked much better.

On my Runcoach training schedule, I added several races and inputted my time of about four hours and fifty minutes for my Denver Colfax Marathon. By adjusting my running schedule with Runcoach and RaceRaves, I got to see some goals met. In the plane at the flight back home, I read magazines and worked on my computer, and the airline hostess was kind and gave me a snack and water. I respected the racing staff to put together a professional race with the main sponsor Cigna that made the race entertaining and socially amusing.

I recently ran a virtual half marathon called the Scary Run hosted by Why Racing and Series Runner, and I received a marathon kit bag and wore a fanny pack with a water bottle holder. I was ready to go and used the restrooms near the beach, saw the scenery, and ran home in time to successfully complete the race.

I ran the 2021 Virtual Cloverdale Kiwanis Vineyard Races Half Marathon on my birthday with a fast pace at the start and placed first to show me that I understand how my body can perform with a race. A goal of flattening my stomach or showing definition in my abs has been rather difficult for me since I weighed an extra one hundred pounds fifteen years ago. Push-ups and exercise did not remove the extra skin or pouch around my stomach area, and it will not naturally go away. A recent CAT scan in December 2021 showed a tiny fat-containing umbilical hernia that was treated through surgery at Kaiser Permanente, which is where I went as a kid and both my parents are members. I'm working toward a proper recovery with no lifting or pulling ten pounds for six weeks and to get more sleep.

The 2021 Two Cities Marathon was in Fresno, California, and I started to prepare by balancing my running, work, rest, and my vision of the race. I choose to drive to the expo instead of flying to save time and money, and the experience of driving differs from flying because I'm in control of the road, and I need to watch the road. Running with joy comes from within and from others, and with a visualization of your goals, you can start to prepare mentally to develop skills to focus on your fitness. The expo had vendors at booths helping me with anything from a chiropractic check to thermo neck exam, and the Central Valley Fit community booth gave me a free water bottle and entrance in a raffle to win a free entry to a 10K race.

I picked up my T-shirt and race bib from another table, and after the expo, I drove to a restaurant to eat a healthy pasta and chicken meal. I drove to my motel, and I managed to get a late checkout because I told the front desk again about my marathon. I went online to work with Uber Eats, and the change of working in Fresno was loved since the customers and restaurants were friendly. The race was cold in the morning, and the weather was foggy. I was shaking a little, but I managed to dress with the short-sleeve shirt the race gave me and shorts of my own. I ran with an eight-minute-per-mile pace at the beginning of the race, and I averaged about eleven minutes per mile.

The Two Cities Marathon course was mostly flat and was sponsored by CalViva, and it started and finished at Clovis Community College. Before the start of the race, I met someone named Sergio that ran the Boston Marathon virtually for the first time, and I learned that it was the first year that was possible, and there is no need to get the fast-qualifying time to qualify. I met various pacers before the race too who saw me on the course and said I was doing a noble job. The weather was very cold in the morning, but I warmed up later and built enough heat to feel healthy at the starting line, and I ran the whole race without eating any protein bars.

The announcer called my name and noticed my achievement, saying, "Ali Mazhin from Rancho Palos Verdes, running for Series Runner, thank you." I received a wonderful finisher's medallion, and many people congratulated me after my race. I relaxed and wanted to recover. I had a pancake breakfast with an ice cream sundae with some other finishers who chatted with me about their successes with pace and time, and we listened to a band play, entertaining music by Journey. I drove safely back home in about five hours, making frequent trips to use the restrooms along the way.

I also finished a Silver Strand 10K in Coronado recently, and I was excited to get more miles completed toward the Series Runner Challenge. I drove to Coronado and parked by the beach, picked up my shirt, raced with others successfully, and got a medal after the finish line. I showered near the beach, and worked with Uber Eats after the run. It was thrilling to feel my efforts worked to deliver pick up food from restaurants and deliver it to customers.

I had a three-mile fun run called the Forty-First Annual Harry Sutter Memorial Turkey Trot in Torrance, on Thanksgiving, which was the night after receiving my COVID-19 booster, and I made it through the tiredness in good heart to enjoy my Thanksgiving dinner.

The 2021 Seattle Amica Marathon was a Series Runner Medal Race and run in person and virtually, and the price of airline tickets was rather high, but my priorities were to prevent injuries and dress warm for the rain. I ran and submitted my virtual Seattle marathon results earlier in the year, and I was one step closer to completing the full marathon in person. The time I spent toward the plane flight, car rental, expo, shopping, and the marathon itself was exciting and rewarding because of achieving my medal and for the scenery in the race.

My flight with Delta Air Lines left on time, and my communication with the airline staff and the passenger right beside me went well. The pilot looked over to the flight attendants and gave instructions after a safe landing.

The Seattle-Tacoma International Airport in Tacoma, Washington, was modern. I let my mom know about my plans for the weekend ahead when I landed, and I took a shuttle to pick up my rental car, and I didn't pay for extra insurance because I have insurance with the Automobile Club of California (AAA). The host hotel for the expo of the Seattle Amica Insurance Marathon was at the Westin Seattle hotel, and I reserved a room ahead of time. The hotel was modern, met my expectations, and had a gym. I took the elevator to the floor to pick up my bib number, and I talked to the race staff about how to get to the starting line, the shuttle times, and other instructions about the race.

After the expo, I drove to a nearby Whole Foods Market for food, and I visited various street fairs that were filled with beautiful lighted Christmas trees. The Whole Foods Market saved me money from paying for meals at the expo or in Seattle restaurants, and I bought organic food on sale for the weekend. I drove to the Westin and parked my car in a nearby area with the smallest charge, and I went to my hotel room, showered, slept, requested a wake-up call, and talked to my mom about getting rest. The shuttle area was downstairs from the expo. I wore the wristband given to me at the expo to go the with a bus, and I met fellow runners that had stories to tell that were thought-provoking.

A firefighter originally from California shared with me about his life and his goals for the race, and I shared to him my expected finish time. He took pictures of me at the starting line, and I smiled to be in the race at the right time and place. Another runner shared that at one time, he was 250 pounds, and running helped him to lose weight and stay fit. The announcer was easygoing and welcomed the runners with a professional commentary that motivated me to run. I started the race in the front, and I was in the lead for a small time for the first time. Many runners caught up to me, including pacers who often told me that I did nice work. I focused on running without injury, and the trees and scenery made me appreciate the environment. I focused on my feet instead of the aches, fractures, or cramps.

The talked with the runners and volunteers to run at a pace near nine minutes per mile while handling the hills well. The race went through the University of Washington and was sponsored by the Amica Insurance, and the university's medicine department helped runners at the stations.

I finished the race and kept a distance after the finish line, and the announcer said, "Ali Mazhin from Palos Verdes." The medal was given to me by the finish line staff. It was beautiful, and it had an improved design from the virtual marathon. I enjoyed the snacks given to me, and I got an Uber ride back to the Westin in Seattle. I was congratulated by the hotel staff upon getting to the hotel, and I talked to my parents and told them my time was actually four hours, seven minutes, and ten seconds.

The experience showed me that I was running races to complete the Series Runner Challenge and to be rewarded later. I updated some of my running apps and websites, and I worked on a Toastmasters speech about my pleasant experience in Seattle.

I registered and completed the Santa Hustle Virtual Marathon, and I ran faster throughout the local beaches and enjoyed the scenery and the day. I ran the Santa to the Sea Half Marathon with Series Runners, and I drove to the race and made it to the shuttles on time and met many people and added miles for my challenge. In the starting line of the race, there was an announcer who talked with passion, and I took a picture with Santa Claus and saw the theme of the run.

The race had many volunteers similar to others, and the course was flat. I kept a nine-minute-per-mile pace, and I was on target. I listened to many bands playing music, and many runners motivated me. I sprinted toward at the finish line and saw runners I met at the starting line. I got a shuttle to pick up my car, and I felt happy to tell my mom about my experience.

Running can let you learn a variety of skills to use in everyday life. The challenges that I have decided to partake leave me with many medals, certificates, achievement, and awards to show. My satisfaction from running is inside of me, and it keeps me looking forward to being a winner and earning a prize. I hope you find my book to inspire you to develop your running in the right direction.

ABOUT THE AUTHOR

Ali Mazhin started to write his book *The Running Journey* in March 2020, and this is his second published book. The first book he wrote was called *Who Is This Person?*, published by New Age World Publishing, first edition, in July 13, 2018. *The Running Journey* differs from his previous book because he chose to make it a purely positive story to motivate people with his running success and to teach people how to train and be safe with their runs. It consists of many experiences that he had in racing events, and he tries to paint a picture of the running world so it's easy to understand and to move the readers.

He took the time to write the book at various places such as at home, on the airplane to races, at hotels, and anywhere he felt safe to do so. He was born in Tehran, Iran, and his parents moved when he was six months old after the Iranian Revolution to the state of Indiana in the United States of America. Four years later, his sister was born in Bloomington, and the family moved to Rolling Hills Estates, California. Two years later, they moved to Rancho Palos Verdes, California, and he continues to live with his parents and considers himself an American because he grew up and went to school in the United States.

He has family and relatives that live and work in Iran and other family and relatives that live throughout the United States. He's traveled many places around the world such as Turkey, Italy, Canada, Spain, and Russia with his parents. He has one job at Ralphs grocery store as a front-end ripper, courtesy clerk, greeter, and combo clerk and another job with Uber Eats as a delivery driver, which keeps him busy and active with the community. He keeps close to his relatives, family, and friends and communicates well with his coworkers daily from

Ralphs and with the customers and merchants he meets through Uber Eats. His father was diagnosed with Parkinson's, Alzheimer's, dementia, and subdural hematoma, and needs care twenty-four hours a day.

He graduated with his undergraduate degree of bachelor of science in finance from California State University Dominguez Hills (CSUDH) in December of 2001. He later graduated his master of business administration (MBA) degree in general business from CSUDH in May of 2017. He worked hard to finish his MBA and is very proud of his achievements, and he considers himself educated and continually learns new things. He enjoys reading, writing, cooking, running, and working two jobs in his spare time.

He has a passion for running races such as 5Ks, half marathons, marathons, ultramarathons, and trail runs, which consist of either virtual or physical races. He travels to various marathons across the United States, from places such as Colorado, Northern California, Southern California, San Diego, Seattle, Washington, San Juan Island, Washington, Park City, Utah, and to San Francisco, California. He enjoys participating and completing various running series or challenges such as the Series Runner Challenge, the Beach Cities Challenge, and the Golden State Challenge. His health is very important for him to maintain, and his diet consists of eggs, fish, chicken, rice, ground turkey, pasta, and other balanced healthy meals. He exercises and runs on his own, with many apps such as the 24 Hour Fitness app called Future, which gives him a personal trainer and several workouts per week with guidance.

He enjoys speaking with Toastmasters International as a member of two clubs, The Health and Wellness Toastmasters and Top Sales. He earned the highest award, the Distinguished Toastmaster Award (DTM), on June 1, 2021; and he's the previous director of Division A3 and the current area director of Division D1, which is an executive position and involves a lot of communication to various clubs. His speaking with Toastmasters improves his confidence as a public speaker, and he participates through Zoom with many clubs as a club coach and member.